When I Die, Take My Panties

When I Die, Take My Panties

Turning Your Darkest Moments into Your Greatest Gifts

JENNIFER COKEN

(P)

When I Die, Take My Panties

Turning Your Darkest Moments into Your Greatest Gifts

© 2017 JENNIFER COKEN.

Published by Persona Publishing.

ISBN 978-0-98337-153-3 paperback
ISBN 978-0-98337-154-0 eBook

Cover Design by:
Rachel Lopez
www.r2cdesign.com

Interior Design by:
Bonnie Bushman
The Whole Caboodle Graphic Design

"Life is not a journey to the grave with the intention of arriving safely in a pretty and well preserved body, but rather to skid in broadside, thoroughly used up, totally worn out, and loudly proclaiming — WOW— What a Ride!"
—Author Unknown

Acknowledgements

There are so many I want to acknowledge for making this book possible. I honestly wasn't sure I'd actually publish. It wasn't that I didn't want to; I was simply "busy" with life. Upon reflection I can now see that I was procrastinating to avoid finally closing this particular chapter of my life. Completion can be confronting – especially when we have grown to be comfortable in the space we are in.

I want to start by thanking my family for supporting me during the time my mom was sick – thank you for your love, your honesty and for listening to so much so many times over. A very special thanks to my aunt and uncle and my dad and stepmom who made a very tough time in my life so much easier knowing that I had you all in my life.

Next I want to thank my writing coach and mentor Kristen Moeller of the company Author Your Brilliance who teased this book out of me as she does for so many writers. Kristen, your unwavering support of this project made me believe in myself in a way that wouldn't have been possible without you! Thank you for believing in me and making it possible to get published.

I want to thank Suzanne Muller-Heinz my friend, fearless writing partner and author of *Lovable*. Suz, you are such a great listener, operate with so much integrity and are so darned determined - you have always been and continue to be an inspiration to me with your success. I also want to thank Linda Hampton and Shoshanna French – both of whom kept reminding me to let go of everything having to be perfect and "just get the book out there." You are both such wise women! Linda, it made such a difference to be with you in your house in Mexico to do the final edit and hone in on the main points of the book. That ten-minute conversation caused all of the pieces to simply fit together.

Thank you Ilene Rosenblum, you literally gave me sanctuary back in 2012 so that I could write the book in the first place. Thank you for your kind and generous heart and for opening your home to me and to Sadie. Thank you Mary Ann Tate for your stellar copy editing and pushing me to read. Thank you to my tight circle of girlfriends who helped me through this difficult period of time – Heather, Beth, Rebecca, Esther, Sierra and Dana. And finally to Sumir – for your final proofread and for relating to the book in a way I hadn't even thought about. You have been and will continue to be such a contribution to my life.

There are so many more people to thank for their contribution to the completion of this book – the Seminar Leader body, staff and Landmark Forum Leader body of Landmark Worldwide; all of my friends and "family" in Denver and my friends and family on the East Coast; and in particular my circle of "witches and warlocks" (you know who you are) that kept me sane along the way.

Finally, I want to thank Werner Erhardt who created the est training back in the day – which I did at the age of 15 at the encouragement of my mom. Having that language in common allowed for so much during the last years of her life. Especially our ability to take all the meaning out of everything we were dealing with and choosing to create our lives and the future moment by moment.

I love you and appreciate each and every one of you.

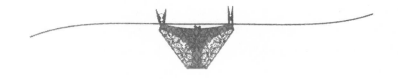

Chapter 1
Death Schmeath

On August 10, 2006 my mom was diagnosed with stage four ovarian cancer. Statistically speaking she had less than an 18% chance of living for five more years. She lived five years, one month and eight days. This is not a story about battling cancer or hope prevailing or even a miracle cure at the end. It is a story of a woman who tap danced her way through chemotherapy, loved her family and friends ferociously, and tried every option she could find to stick around as long as possible.

This is the story of a woman who went from being a logical teacher and scientist who did not believe that there was anything more than what she could see, touch or feel, to being a woman who believed there was a divine spirit in each of us and accepted that her cancer was part of her journey in this lifetime.

But mostly it is my story about the lessons I had throughout my life that I had no idea were preparing me for living with the uncertainty of Mom's diagnosis. There were situations and circumstances that happened before, during and after Mom's diagnosis and death that led me to a real place of peace within a year of her passing – a genuine place of peace where I could authentically say I wouldn't have changed anything.

During the last five years of Mom's life, there were times when I was strong, like the time we were searching for an experimental drug that was the one hope of saving Mom's life, or when I was helping her visualize a healthy future; or we were planning her seventieth birthday party. Then there were the times (mostly) when I was terrified, frozen by my fears, trying to will any negative thoughts out of my mind lest they take root and become real. Then there were those times that I was just plain good old fashioned pissed off – fuck cancer. At four o'clock every afternoon my family and I would stop everything we were doing to give cancer the "bird" – SCREW YOU CANCER!!! We didn't ask for you. We don't want you. And quite honestly there is only so "Zen" I can be about watching someone I love waste away to an unseen force that we had no control of no matter how hard we tried to convince ourselves that we did.

Toward the end when Mom called to tell me the doctors had told her that there was nothing more they could do, reality set in. My mom was going to die. That was the predictable future from the beginning but it was only in those last few months that I finally came to believe that future would be real. People would say to me, "Jennifer, you didn't think she would live, did you?" Yes, I did. I really did. I believed my mom when she said, "I can live with this just the way people do with diabetes." I believed because anything less felt like giving up, copping out, and throwing in the towel. Anything less and I'd have to start imagining life without my mom. Anything less and I'd have to admit that I was scared of her death as well as my own.

I never would have admitted I was afraid of death; I just didn't think about it. Who honestly does unless you've gone through something like this or another terrible trauma when you've come face to face with it? When people asked how I felt about Mom dying I'd say cavalierly "Well we're all gonna die one day." My mom and stepdad Max, who was thirteen years her senior, used to send me quarterly updates to their wills, notes about where their safe-deposit box was, a listing of their investments, and a reminder that I was second in line as the executor of my mom's will so I should pay attention. Each time the envelope arrived I would dutifully throw it into the fireproof box without opening it. If they asked if I had read it, I'd lie. I just didn't see what was so important about all of that. What's the big deal? I never imagined my mom dying. She was a health nut.

In 1976, after she and my dad got divorced, she became a hippie vegetarian. She went to Europe for a month. She bought Birkenstock's and sundresses while she was there. She read *Diet for a Small Plant.* She began making her own yogurt and bread. She developed a new habit of speed walking around the neighborhood at five-thirty every morning. She took so many supplements during the course of a day I wondered how she got anything accomplished.

I hid my fear well. I prided myself on being a bit of a badass. I'd jumped out of an airplane once. I'd ridden my bike thousands of miles from Fairbanks to Anchorage, Alaska with cracked ribs and from Montreal to Portland, Maine with a torn tendon. I did nine rides from North Carolina to Washington, DC in extreme heat – one ride dehydrated me so badly I needed an IV, but I got up the next day, got on the bike and did it again. I'd performed stand-up comedy many times as the only female in the line-up and kept going through deafening silence broken only by someone in the back clearing his or her throat.

The month before Mom died I did my very first paid comedy gig to an audience of 75, a two-woman show that we called "Hot Chicks with Brains." In it, I used humor as a way to talk about Mom's death and what I was going through. It was hard to write the material and scarier to perform it, but none of those events or any others in my life took the kind of courage I had to tap into for dealing with the inevitable—living life without Mom.

Mom's death from ovarian cancer was, for me, much like kids who find out that Santa Claus isn't real. (I'm Jewish and although we had a Christmas tree I was very clear Santa Claus was about as real as Hanukkah Charlie.) Her death altered my view of myself and what I thought I could achieve. Before she died, I believed there was nothing I couldn't make happen. In fact, I prided myself on making things happen, especially under pressure. I'd been a grassroots organizer for nearly twenty-five years. While I hadn't won every single campaign I'd ever worked on, you bet we had made a lot of noise and gotten the right people's attention. In my world, when I said something was going to happen, it happened.

But this time I failed.

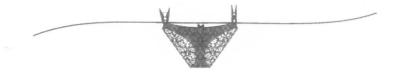

Chapter 2
Please, Take My Panties

From time to time as people learned about my mother's condition, because I openly talked about it, inevitably the following would happen. Someone, usually another woman, would come up to me with eyes a bit downcast, put her hand on my arm and say in a hushed tone, "I heard about your mother. I know that this may not make sense now, but it will be the most beautiful time of your lives." All I could think at that very moment was, "Fuck. You."

It wasn't beautiful to see Mom's collarbone and ribs sticking out through her skin in her final days. It wasn't beautiful to watch her belly get bigger and bigger until she literally looked like she was nine months pregnant. She would stand up and start scratching like a pregnant woman whose skin had expanded to accommodate the growing life inside. But this "pregnancy" was sucking the life out of her.

It wasn't beautiful watching her moan in her wheelchair in the emergency room because she'd been throwing up all day and couldn't keep her pain medication down. It wasn't beautiful watching her dry heave, bent over in pain while waving my stepfather and me away because she couldn't stand to be touched as we attempted to rub her back to soothe her. How she smelled wasn't beautiful. I walked into her home about a month before she died and I could smell the wasting away of a body. I could smell death nearby. She couldn't help it and it didn't matter anyway. It was painful. It sucked. It tore my heart out that I couldn't stop nature from taking its course. I couldn't come up with a different ending.

In the end my mother asked me to make sure she had a beautiful death. "I've had a beautiful life, I want a beautiful death," she said. I knew she didn't mean a pretty one because she, above anyone, knew how she looked. (She had confided in me that she had stopped looking in the mirror a long time ago.) What she meant was she wanted to enjoy every moment that she had left, just like she had enjoyed every moment of living up to that point. In her final days, my mom was at peace with dying because she knew she had tried every possible way to prolong her life.

She gave everything to her family—figuratively and literally. The final week I was with her, about a month before she entered hospice, we went through every closet and every drawer in her dresser so she could give me the things she thought I would like: some jewelry, a formal gown, and a special shawl. "Here, take my panties," she said. She held up about two-dozen pairs of Hanky Panky thong underwear. "They are $20 each and I've barely worn them. Will you take them? They shouldn't go to waste." I shrugged, smiled, and told her I would.

She had always been a very practical person and I couldn't say no. I remembered a time in high school when I was walking with her and happened to nonchalantly chuck six pennies over the side of bridge onto an embankment below. "What did you just throw?" she asked. "I threw six pennies, they aren't worth much." "Ninety four more cents and you've got a dollar, go get them." I thought she was crazy but she stood there until I climbed through the fence and walked down to get them. I resented every moment but that memory stuck with me my whole life. I shouldn't have been surprised because I remember a story about the first year she and my dad were married. They told each other they were not going to get each other gifts because they were so poor. But my mom, ever the saver, saved up every extra quarter she had and bought my dad a new blue bathrobe for $25. He was shocked and embarrassed he hadn't done the same. That was my mom though, always a saver and always taking really good care of her possessions so that they lasted a long time. Good qualities that I've tried to embrace during my life – sometimes successfully and sometimes not.

And for all of those people who told me this would be the most beautiful time of my life? Thank you. I know you meant well. You had gone through what I was going through and your words were designed to comfort me. I just wasn't ready to hear them so I am not bitter or angry (even though each time, admittedly, I did kinda want to punch you in the throat). In the end you were right. In many ways those five years, one month and eight days wound up being some of the most beautiful moments of our lives.

It was beautiful, and it was hard and sad and funny. I've never wept so much. I've never been so angry or so desperate. I've never loved so much. I've never laughed so hard nor shared so much. I walked away with a new heart, a new vision for life, and a new experience of the world.

In the end, as my mother's voice was silenced, I walked away with a new voice of my own.

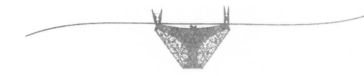

Chapter 3
Are You Willing To Fail Spectacularly?

I moved to Colorado in 2004 to follow my heart. I had met and fallen in love with a park ranger in the fall of 2002. Tim was in law enforcement; a "man's man" as they say. He rode a Harley and seemed able to fix anything. I remember the first time we met he was wearing leather chaps and Wranglers and looked just like a young Kris Kristofferson. As I watched his butt in those jeans, I leaned over to my friend and whispered: "I'm gonna ride that guy out of here." I was smitten.

We had had a long-distance relationship for a year and a half. We spoke daily and emailed each other constantly. I helped him move from a job in Utah to a better one in Colorado. At one point while we were lying in bed together in his cabin in the middle of nowhere Colorado, I summoned up all my courage and told him I loved him. "I know. I can see it in your eyes," he responded. Not the response I was hoping for but at least I told him how I felt. I had faith that he was falling for me, too—even if he didn't say so. I mean he was the strong silent type after all.

Tim told me from the beginning he'd never move east of the Mississippi. "Too many people," he'd say. I had a great life in DC and wasn't planning to move anytime soon, either. We talked about the 2,000-mile distance and agreed that our connection was so rare that we would take things one day at a time and figure it out as we went along.

The Universe has a funny way of smacking you on the butt sometimes. Out of nowhere I was laid off because the organization I worked for had run out of funding. Tim had already moved to Colorado. I had no job and I'd always wanted to live there. Seemed like a good time to move, no? Whoa. Wait a minute. What? I was considering moving 2,000 miles away from everyone and everything I was comfortable with for a man? Me? Ms. Independent? Nah…but that is exactly where my brain went as I walked down the street in the summer sunshine after getting the bad news from my boss.

On one hand my life in DC was really full and wonderful. I had a great social network revolving around cycling. I had a great group of close friends. I had been mentored by some really powerful women who helped me become a go-to person in the fields of fundraising and designing youth service programs. I couldn't have been happier, with one exception. I was not in the deliciously romantic, make-your-toes-curl, head-over-heels, passionately loving relationship that I'd dreamed of for a very long time.

"What if Tim is the one and I don't go for it because I'm comfortable here and if truth be told, too darned scared to go for it? I imagined myself at ninety, sitting in my rocking chair on the porch of an old-age home, looking out at the trees. There I'd sit, a non-filter Camel cigarette in one hand, dentures in a glass next to me so they didn't get tobacco stained, the arthritic knuckles of my other hand curled around a glass of good, single-malt scotch, fuzzy blanket tucked in around my painfully thin legs as I sat in my wheelchair next to my best friend Tammy.

"You remember Tim?" I'd shout.

"Whaaat?" Tammy bellowed back.

"Tim, the park ranger, the one in Colorado," I'd reply.

"Oh yeah, him. You really loved him once. What ever happened to him?" she'd say.

"No idea. Lost touch with him. Maybe I should've moved to Colorado."

I think when I'm ninety all I will have is time, time to sit and think about my life, the people in it, the people I wronged, the chances I never took, the people I loved and those who loved me. I didn't want to be ninety and regret that I didn't move because I was too afraid.

As I thought about my life in DC, I realized that, though I was happy, I was also complacent in a weird way. I had taken a lot of risks since arriving 11 years earlier including quitting my Capitol Hill job to start my own consulting firm with Arianna Huffington as my first client – giving up a 9 to 5 job with no steady income had required a total leap of faith on my part. But since that time I had started a number of successful non-profits that were impacting the city in really amazing ways. I was proud of those achievements but can I admit to you that I was bored? I just didn't feel challenged anymore. I was doing the same things with the same people in the same ways.

I did love my life. I had learned how to ride my bike hundreds of miles over a few days to raise money for charity – this from someone who hadn't ridden a bike more than five or six miles when she started. My dad had given me an old bike of his and was ecstatic that his daughter was taking up his hobby. I went from not being able to walk after a training ride because my legs were so sore to leading training rides for new riders and encouraging women new to the sport. The friends I made were the largest part of my social circle in DC. We planned weekend rides, we spent holidays together, and we had each other's backs. I loved those people; they were my family.

There was absolutely nothing wrong with my life and I was really happy. Many people would have been satisfied, and I was, in most aspects. Yet, there was one challenge I had never undertaken—the challenge of giving my heart over to someone when I had no guarantee of an outcome. Not even one "I love you, too." Truth be told, when I called Tim to suggest I move to Colorado, he freaked out. He didn't want me to be mad at him if things didn't work out. "I don't want that responsibility," he said. I understood where he was coming from but this move was more about getting out of my own comfort zone and being willing to confront myself and my beliefs than it was about putting any pressure on him to commit. I explained that to him and he did understand. "If I chose to move, that is my choice, and I'm not going to blame you for anything," I assured him.

I had a lot to think about. Should I take the risk? Between you and me I had always ridiculed other women who followed their boyfriends from place to place, or wives whose lives had revolved around their husbands and families. I hated those women who forgot about their friends when they got into a relationship. I vowed to never do anything like that. I judged women who did that as weak. I thought that they thought loving someone that much meant you had to sacrifice your own dreams for theirs. Hell if I was going to do that for any man.

But wait. Maybe, just maybe, I was wrong. What if the strength I was so proud of had me keeping walls up? What if being vulnerable enough to give your whole heart to someone and sacrificing your "you" for the possibility of a "we" was one of the most powerful actions a person could take? How much courage and audacity would a person have to have to do something like that? That kind of a bold, courageous action could come with a surprise ending – or the whole thing could go down in flames. But I already knew the predictable future if I took no action at all. I talked this over with a good friend who took me on a field trip to Theodore Roosevelt Island just outside Washington, DC. There he shared with me one of his favorite Teddy Roosevelt quotes:

"It is not the critic who counts; not the man who points out how the strong man stumbles, or where the doer of deeds could have done them better. The credit belongs to the man who is actually in the arena, whose face is marred by dust and sweat and blood; who strives valiantly; who errs, who comes short again and again, because there is no effort without error and shortcoming; but who does actually strive to do the deeds; who knows great enthusiasms, the great devotions; who spends himself in a worthy cause; who at the best knows in the end the triumph of high achievement, and who at the worst, if he fails, at least fails while daring greatly, so that his place shall never be with those cold and timid souls who neither know victory nor defeat."

I read the quote and sat quietly trying to absorb the lesson he was trying to teach me. Then he said "Are you going to sit on the sidelines because you are afraid, or are you willing to fail spectacularly? What's the worst that can happen? You can always come back."

I looked into his eyes and was silent for a few moments. The guy in front of me had been a Navy Seal, he had been in more life and death situations than I could ever imagine or would ever hear about. This was not a life or death situation but in that moment it felt like it was life or death for the expansion of my very own soul. Tears formed in the corners of my eyes and one started rolling down my cheek. I was shaking because I had never stood on this precipice before.

"I am willing to fail spectacularly," I whispered.

"Good girl," he said.

That moment is one I will never forget. That conversation on that sunny afternoon on Roosevelt Island with a friend led me to sell everything lock, stock and barrel and move to Colorado. The willingness to fail spectacularly became a mantra for my life. That man changed my perspective on life in that one instant – it's a moment I'm forever grateful for and one I'll never forget.

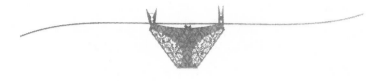

Chapter 4
One Stick Shift That Changed The World

Tim came to my going away party, poor thing. My DC friends grilled him about how he was going to make certain I stayed in touch with them. I was surprised that they asked that question because I knew (and Tim knew) I was so stubborn that no one could make me do anything I didn't want to do. Conversely, my friends were such a big part of my life, asking that question seemed ridiculous to me. "How could I not stay in touch with them?" I thought to myself.

I dropped Tim off at the airport at Terminal A to return to Colorado and swung around to Terminal C to pick up my mom. God love her. She was taking time off work to drive across the country with my two cats and me. I was surprised she was willing to go with me. Mom just didn't seem like the type to want to go on a cross-country adventure.

However, I had learned through the years never to underestimate her, like the time I was running my first political campaign as part of my master's program. Mom came down for the Fourth of July weekend to see what I was doing as campaign manager for a state representative race.

There I was, gingerly placing the candidate and her husband in two unsecured lawn chairs in the back of a pick-up truck as part of the ride in the local Fourth of July parade. The volunteer who loaned us the truck had already taken off to go join the Shriners. It was time to line up for the parade, so I hoisted myself into the cab to drive to the starting line. I looked down and realized the truck had a manual transmission. Crap, I had never learned to drive a stick.

"It's a stick shift. I can't drive it. Who can?" I asked the crowd of supporters, the only people I would trust with such precious cargo.

Everyone stared back at me blankly. None of them could drive a stick. We were in the middle of Southern Ohio, for gosh sakes—farm country. These people had grown up on tractors, hadn't they? No one could drive a stick shift? Double Crap. I was sunk. I hadn't thought about this possible disaster.

Then from behind the group came a quiet voice: "I can drive a stick shift." And like the Red Sea parting for Moses, the volunteers opened up a pathway for my 47-year old Mom.

"You can drive a stick shift?" I asked incredulously?

"Yep, used to drive a big yellow school bus for the local school district after college," she answered.

I smiled broadly, as much pleasantly surprised by her as I was laughing at myself, and shook my head. I bet there is a lot more to my mom than just this one surprise, I thought. I had no idea how true this statement would be until her death 24 years later.

So we drove from Washington, DC to Colorado through four days of snowstorms, freezing temperatures and a few hints of sunlight. We passed the time taking turns holding my nervous cat Sadie on our laps. Her husky brother Junior, weighing in at 16 pounds, was happy to sleep the entire time. I'm sure if I'd had a tiny HDTV switched on to football he would have leaned back with one paw rubbing his enormous belly, the claws on his other paw sunk deep into a can of Pabst Blue Ribbon Beer. Sadie was another story. She got carsick very easily and was a bit of a princess. Whenever I had to take her somewhere, she would meow continuously and began to foam at the mouth from her nausea. Normally, I would just shush her while driving because the distances were short. But that didn't work on a 2,000-mile road trip. The vet had given me some medication to sedate her but we couldn't get it in her mouth without being bitten. When we did succeed, she just threw it back up. The only way she would stay quiet was if we swaddled her in a blanket and took turns holding in her on our lap. For over 1,600 miles, we held the swaddled baby-cat and Mom never said a word about it. She just did what worked for me and for Sadie. That was Mom. She always did for others, even if it meant giving up her own comfort.

By the time we rolled into Denver at seven in the evening after four days of driving, we were shot. Tim was meeting us later with air mattresses, extra blankets and towels. Our welcoming committee consisted of a good friend and her two-year-old daughter wearing a fantastic pair of hot pink sequined cowboy boots holding out a plate of chocolate covered strawberries. "For you!" she looked up at me with her enormous crystal-blue eyes, chocolate already covering her face. "You want one? I do," she said as she picked up a strawberry and started to rub it around her mouth. "Mmmm, you should try it."

So I did. I joined Dawn in her two-year old delight as we walked into the apartment building. At that point the apartment was completely devoid of furniture. The moving truck wouldn't arrive for at least another two days. As we set down our suitcases, there was a knock at the door. There stood Tim, his head cocked to one side, his blue eyes lit with excitement at seeing me. "Hello Darlin', welcome to Colorado," he said as he wrapped me in a bear hug. He had not only brought air mattresses, bedding, sheets and towels, but a beautiful bouquet of flowers and a vase to go with it. I thought: this may be one of the best decisions I've ever made.

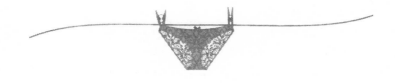

Chapter 5
The Ronald Reagan Years

Although I'd spent most of my 25-year career working in politics in one form or another, I came into it by accident. I graduated high school when I was 16 years old – the result of a combination of skipping second grade and having a birthday in August. High school was difficult for me. My classes bored me, and I wasn't very interested in applying myself, anyway. I never felt like I really fit in anywhere, so I kept to my small circle of girlfriends and spent a lot of time at the library reading. Mom and I talked and agreed that I should wait a year before going to college so I could save some money. I found out years later that she was worried about my ability to cope with college life and wanted me to be more mature before venturing out into the world.

I always wanted to be an actor. My family had been part of a local community theater for years. I had dreams about living and working in New York City and being like one of those kids in *Fame*. So we agreed. If that was what I really wanted, I would wait a year, work, save up money and apply to acting schools. It was great, that is until all my friends started making plans to go to college. At some point my best friend and I hatched a plan to go to the local state university. I told my mom I'd go for one year and then switch to a small liberal arts college to pursue my acting dream.

I was sixteen when I started freshman orientation and seventeen-and-a-day when I started classes. I had most of the freshman classes: Sociology 101, Psychology 101, French, Trig and American Political Science. I was just biding my time by taking general courses that would be transferable once I decided on a good liberal arts college. Little did I know, that first day of political science would change my life forever.

My professor was fascinating and brilliant. He had just started a new Master of Political Science Program for the school with a Certification in Political Campaign Management. I had paid little attention to politics before I walked into his classroom, but I was hooked after just one class. He made politics come alive. He talked a mile a minute and waved his hands and asked us for our opinions. He didn't scoff if we didn't have the right answer. He told us why following politics mattered, why we mattered and that every citizen had an obligation to get involved in their local community. He made me believe that I could make a difference in society if I wanted to and took action.

I walked up to him at the end of the hour and declared right then and there that I would be a participant in his graduate school program. At age 17, I suddenly had my entire life mapped out in front of me. Forget acting. I'd finish my BA, go for my MA and manage political campaigns. I'd be clever and famous and get Presidents elected, just like Richard Gere in the movie *Power*. That was going to be me one day—

crafting smart radio and television commercials and advising powerful men. (I knew of few women in politics at that time.) I'd be sought after around the country.

So I spent my undergraduate years immersed in political science and political philosophy courses. I was involved in the Democratic Club, and when my cohorts and I decided that club was too conservative, we started our own Democratic Alternative Club. I worked at the Center for Peaceful Studies, learned about the Kent State shootings and studied the history of non-violent protest. Finally, something had captured my imagination and I was involved in campus activities in a way that I'd never been in high school.

Graduate school was like a dream come true. The courses were difficult but the people in my program were brilliant. They were much older because they had all come from the workforce so they had real life stories to tell. They were as enamored with the political process as I was, and we spent many nights drinking beer and pretending we had all the answers to the world's political problems. We were going to change the world one campaign at a time. Each of us was required to run an actual campaign as part of our curriculum. My master's thesis was a 100-page campaign plan for a State Representative race in Southern, Ohio. I packed my bags and drove south, having no idea that the next seven months would drastically change the direction of my life.

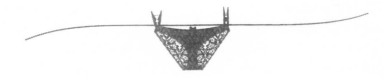

Chapter 6
Sometimes There Are No Choices

I t was an unseasonably warm, sunny, Ohio day in September 1986. I was driving my new car, a 1980 Chevy Impala, a gift from my parents for my upcoming graduation from graduate school. A huge bronze machine, it had mag wheels and its own stereo system complete with tape deck—now that was fancy. The bronze exterior matched the leather interior. I dubbed the car "The Library" because it was eerily quiet as I drove, which was in sharp contrast to the two beater cars I had driven during college. I had the windows wide open and the stereo cranked playing "Walk This Way" by Run D.M.C. and Aerosmith. I was singing along at the top of my lungs with two volunteers in the backseat. I was 21 years old. I was running a political campaign. I was on top of my game.

"Go straight through the next light?" I queried Melinda, one of the high school student-volunteers in the back seat.

"Yep, keep going straight, I'll tell you where to turn," she replied.

I followed the green arrows pointing downward at the lanes in the road and avoided the red "x's" marking those lanes that were going in the opposite direction during rush hour. My mom had taught me to drive during rush hour in Cleveland, Ohio so I was used to following those signs. As I headed into the intersection going about thirty miles an hour, I noticed a car coming down the hill from my left and assumed they would stop because I had the right of way.

Problem was I didn't have the right of way. I may have been following those green arrows, but I had just blown through a red light without realizing it. They didn't stop because they assumed I would – that is what red lights are for right? Time slowed down as I watched our two cars make full-on contact in the middle of the intersection. Their front end slammed into my driver's side door causing my car to do a few 360's. We all started screaming and the car finally stopped. My hands gripped the steering wheel at 2:00pm and 10:00pm, my arms outstretched, locked in place as if rigor mortis had set in days earlier. I unclenched my jaw and looked into the back seat.

The girls were crying but seemed fine. They didn't seem to have any broken bones or massive wounds. The impact of the crash had been so hard that the bottom half of the seat had torn away from the top. My left front wheel was collapsed in on itself; the hood was crumpled and steam rose up from the engine. The car was totaled. My parents were going to kill me.

I then remembered the other car. I looked over to my right and the other car was nose first in a ditch with the front end crunched up around a telephone pole. Other cars had stopped and someone was helping the female driver from the car. She was screaming and moaning in pain. "Please God, let them be okay," I pleaded silently. I got out of the car and started walking over. Someone put their arm around me to steady me as my legs buckled. They told me to sit down and that help was on its way. They put a blanket around my shoulders as I slid to the ground.

The EMTs came and attended to all of us, taking us to a local hospital. Thankfully none of us were hurt very badly. The other driver suffered from muscle strain in her back. Thankfully my insurance covered all of her hospital bills, the physical therapy she needed to receive to alleviate the pain, and all of the damage to her car. I had slight bruising and one of the volunteers had somehow cut her earlobe. The three of us were more scared than hurt. Friends came to pick us up and take us home.

I'd had the car for less than a month. When I called my insurance company, they reminded me that I had transferred the liability insurance but not the collision insurance to the new car because I didn't have a lot of money at the time. I was waiting on my first paycheck to have the money for the monthly premium to increase the insurance. I had really screwed up. I had no money. My parents had no extra money. Now I had no car and needed one to get around. What the heck was I to do?

One of my closest friends in grad school, Walt, happened to be running a campaign less than an hour away. He came to get me and took me back to his house for dinner and a few much-needed beers so we could discuss my options. In the end, he generously loaned me $300 to buy a used car from the junkyard where my car had been towed. He also agreed to take a look at the car to make sure it was worth buying.

We went over to the junkyard one weekend and met with Frank, the junkyard owner. Frank looked like he was straight out of Central Casting: short, bow-legged and wearing the same dirty John Deere hat every time I saw him. He had a permanent toothpick dangling from the corner of his mouth. His face and hands were rough from driving trucks, managing the family farm and running a junkyard on the side. He was never without a greasy towel hanging from the back pocket of his Wranglers that slapped against his thigh as he used his crowbar to free a part from a junked car for a waiting customer.

When I showed up to check on my car a few weeks earlier, he had chuckled.

"Where's your crutches, girl?" Frank asked.

"Don't have any," I replied softly looking at him out of the corner of my eye.

"The other people survive?"

"Yep, all of us," I replied wincing at his question. How much of a jerk did he think I was?

"Sorry didn't mean to offend, just the last time I saw a car this bad I had to wipe some unidentifiable goop off the seats because it smelled during the hot months. I got cars that stay on this lot for years. I couldn't let it get baked into the leather," he explained.

I shuddered at that conversation and tuned in again to Walt. He had finished looking the car over and told me it was worth it, but needed repairs. He would help me with the minor ones, but the major things would have to be done elsewhere. I had no idea how I would afford those repairs let alone how I'd repay him for the car. I wasn't getting paid for the campaign and had no money in savings. My folks didn't have a lot either and after totaling the car they were still paying on; I couldn't bring myself to go to them. What was I going to do?

"Hey, what do you think?" Walt asked me as we stood next to my "new" car.

"Huh?"

"Girl, pay attention," Frank never called me by my name. He always referred to me as "Girl" or "The Girl" if he referenced me while I was in the same room.

"I said I'd teach you how to do the work on your car right here. We'll pull parts from the other junked cars and you can work off the parts and labor by helping me behind the counter. But you gotta do the work on the car yourself. I'll make certain you do it right, but you might have to do it two or three times."

I looked at Walt and shrugged my shoulders. What other options did I have?

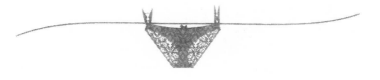

Chapter 7
Tenacious Jen

I spent the next several months working mornings in Frank's junkyard pulling parts for customers and working on my car. I'd get up at four a.m. and drive to Frank's, he'd buy me breakfast since he knew I was broke, and we'd get to the shop by five a.m. I'd wait on customers until eight, shower, and then head over to campaign headquarters by nine. The store was filled with rows and rows of metal shelves housing parts for vehicles going back 20 years or more. He was known for his variety of American made parts and he used every inch of that cavernous space to its fullest advantage. Dirt and grime from years of exhaust and dust covered the boxes and I spent hours inhaling those tiny particles and attempting to keep my nails clean so I could look a bit respectable later on.

Frank would get a kick out of leaving me behind the counter when the big burly guys came in.

"Where's Frank?" they'd ask.

"The Girl's gotcha," he'd shout from the back.

They'd look at me from head to toe, lingering for a moment on my breasts, not in a sexual way but just trying to comprehend that this thing with boobs knew what she was doing around cars, trucks and parts. Frank left me to figure things out by myself, including searching for parts on cars in the junkyard when a customer couldn't afford the new one. He'd watch me trekking through the overgrown lot for ten minutes, tops, before I'd hear him bellow.

"Girl? Whatcha doin'? You know that ain't a Ford. Look at the way the headlights are mounted, that's a Chrysler, the Ford is next to it." I learned quickly.

By eight, the morning rush was over. All the guys who owned repair shops in town had come and gotten what they needed and my replacement had come in.

By nine a.m. I was having a second breakfast, this time with the candidate, her husband and her eight children in their farmhouse on the edge of town. She was a secretary at the local university and was challenging a 30-year Republican incumbent in the Bible Belt. She had protested the Vietnam War in her younger, hippie days, which her opponent seized upon and made into a campaign theme that caught on down in the southern reaches of the state. We had a slim chance, but that chance came from the fact that the university population made up a large portion of the voters in the area. We just had to get our message to enough of them, enough times.

I spent the days campaigning with the candidate and the evenings staffing her at events. On weekends we knocked on doors and attended every summer fair possible in Southern Ohio. By the end of summer, I had become a funnel cake connoisseur and could pick out the winner of the 4-H pig from 100 feet away. When I wasn't working there, I'd be back at the shop with my car up on the lift replacing the brakes or rebuilding the carburetor. On my fourth try rebuilding the carburetor, Frank finally told me what I was doing wrong:

"You just flipped this gasket, Girl. See, flip it over and the put the screws back on."

I knew he was teaching me many valuable lessons, but sometimes I wanted things to be easy and for him to just give me the answer. Nope, this was the summer I was to learn the real meaning of the old adage "practice makes perfect," not to mention finding wells of patience I never knew I had and the ability to follow through and not give up when it looked like the deck was stacked against me.

Frank had a huge heart. He was the last person I saw before I headed back north after losing the election 48 to 52 percent. He knew I was still broke. As we said goodbye, he hugged me hard and then slipped me a $20 while he gave my hand a goodbye shake.

"You can pay me back later," he whispered.

I have never forgotten his generosity during those difficult months. Both he and Walt instilled in me a tenacity I didn't know I had. I learned how to look at any situation as a problem that could be solved rather than something as a thing too big to tackle. Those life lessons were well worth the adventure and the black boogers I blew out of my nose every evening.

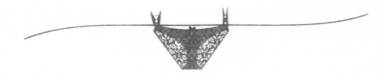

Chapter 8
Turning Myself Inside Out

While we lost the election by four percentage points, many said we did a great job given the demographic make-up of the state. As I drove north toward Cleveland, I realized losing the election wasn't the problem. Losing my idealism was.

I had been on one singular path since my freshman year: move to Washington, DC, and work in the political establishment on Capitol Hill. My final semester in college I participated in a program where I lived and interned in DC. As part of a final requirement, I had to write a 60-page paper. I examined the influence of media on policy and interviewed Members of Congress about the role they thought media played in their decisions. I'd meet with them on the hill then go to the

Library of Congress to transcribe my notes. I bought popsicles from a tiny stand known only to those who used the underground tunnels. I couldn't wait to move back there.

Then the reality of running an actual campaign set in. Every candidate needed money to run a campaign; that was a given. We were pursuing a tiny little state rep seat that wasn't on anyone's radar screen. The folks higher up had their financial priorities already mapped out and all of the Political Action Committees had turned us down. So we relied on our volunteers to help us raise money. I was proud that one massive garage sale netted $7,000. But that would only allow us to contact, maybe, half of our voters one time and we needed to reach out to everyone roughly three to eight times before Election Day. We were cutting corners everywhere we could, but for a bare bones campaign we needed to raise roughly $80,000.

We were especially happy the day the Speaker of the Ohio House of Representatives gave the candidate a check for five figures—all done legally, of course, and with the implicit understanding that, if elected, my candidate would adopt the Speaker's agenda. After all, isn't that how politics works? Our Finance Director happily took the check and deposited it in our ever-dwindling bank account. Yet, I was devastated.

I knew my candidate was squeaky clean and had high moral standards, but what if she had to vote against her conscience because the Speaker asked her to? Would she? I didn't think so but the fact that I had to even consider the question bothered me. What did I really expect? After all, what the heck was the movie *Power* all about anyway but power and the way that power corrupts people and their ideals? I didn't like it, but I understood. I'd spent six years on one, and only one, trajectory. Now I didn't like what I saw. Could I live with the reality of politics?

When I returned to campus to finish up my last few classes, I met with my advisor. She was the chair of the political science department and founder of our women's studies program. I had taken either a political philosophy class or women's studies class from her every semester for four years. She taught me to think and write critically and I found myself confident in my abilities around her. I explained my existential crisis to her. Without batting an eye, she said: "Have you ever thought about working for a grassroots organization that works on issues on the ground by going and talking to voters one on one? There are three interviewing on campus next week." I hadn't considered it, but after doing some research, each organization was doing great things to solve some important social problems, like ending poverty and protecting the environment. I thought I could go to sleep at night working for one of them. I interviewed with both and eventually decided to take a job with the group that paid the highest salary. I was going to make $11,000 a year with my Master's degree. Whoopee. Well, I'd never get rich, but I figured I could live with myself.

That's how I went from having a dream to working inside the beltway to becoming a rabble-rousing game-changer from the outside. I went from my graduate school focus on electoral politics to twenty years of organizing communities around environmental issues to protect the land, air and water. I didn't skip a beat. I didn't look back. I didn't beat myself up. I just beat up the "system." I felt justified for thumbing my nose at the establishment and felt at home knocking on people's doors seven days a week and asking them for money to fund campaigns to save the New Jersey coastline and reduce toxic pollutants from the myriad of chemical plants there. I was at home sleeping on people's floors and living out of my suitcase as I traveled around the country. I was justified representing the "little" people, as it were. I was proud to be a community organizer and I was damned good at my job. The time I spent in Ohio had taught me to be like a pit-bull on a pork chop for causes I believed in.

Eventually I did wind up moving to DC to start a non-profit for a couple of Members of Congress. I was working on welfare reform in the early 1990s when Newt Gingrich and the Republican Party took over the majority in the House. We worked to protect nutrition programs for children, for families and the elderly and we developed leadership programs for youth. I then ran my own consulting firm teaching local community groups how to raise money. I eventually returned to where my heart was—protecting the environment. It was during that time that I met my park ranger Tim, fell in love, and moved to Colorado to follow my heart.

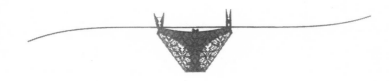

Chapter 9
Jumping Back into the Fray

When I arrived in Colorado in January of 2004 I had no job, a handful of contacts from friends, and a little money in savings that could get me through a few months. I really didn't know what I wanted to do next – stay with non-profits or go back into politics? I decided it was a good time to spend a weekend participating in a personal growth and development course that I hoped would give me some clarity. That experience wound up transforming my life.

I had taken this type of course before, so I knew I was in for a wild ride. I walked in wanting certainty about my next direction and walked out leaving a bunch of career baggage at the door. I went from being stuck and righteous in my disillusionment with the political system to recognizing that twenty years earlier when I had been running my first political campaign, what actually had happened was that the Speaker of the House gave my candidate some money. Period. That was a fact. Everything else that followed was simply my opinion and judgments about what I thought might happen. I found lots and lots of people who agreed with my assessment. At the end of the day, we lost the campaign because we lost the campaign. I never "had to" leave politics as my "moral compass" told me I had to do. No in fact, I could have stuck with politics all along the way. I never had to give up my dream, but I did give up my dream.

By the end of that powerful weekend, my dream to not only be engaged with electoral politics but to run for public office was reignited with a ferocity I hadn't felt since my college years. I decided I would run for office and gave myself a deadline—by 2010—and told the other participants in the course. These were people who I would be seeing regularly as we continued our training, so I knew if I told them, they would hold me to account for what I promised.

My job search took on a new life after that weekend. I started networking and met with 47 people during the month of February. By the end of the month I took a job as the political director for a Member of Congress. Thus began my journey of becoming embedded in local Colorado Democratic politics—something I had never done before. I went from that job to working for the Speaker and Majority Leader of the State House of Representatives, to being elected as the Chair of the County Democratic Party, and to debating the opposition on MSNBC during the Presidential election in 2008. I helped form an organization dedicated to raising money to elect local women candidates to build a bench for future female leadership in the state. In 2010, I kept my promise to run for office largely because so many of the people from that course had become friends and kept asking, "When's your election?"

It also didn't take me long after that weekend to figure out that Tim and I were not going to work out as I thought. We shared a lot of the same values. We had great conversation and loved to laugh together but whatever had happened in his love life before I came on the scene seemed to have a grip on him. At times he was distant, and those times occurred more and more frequently. I felt like I was doing all the work and knew I couldn't make him love me. I didn't realize how hard I had been working at the relationship until that March.

I remember the night it hit me, it was the day before the St. Paddy's Day parade, which was my first big event with the Congresswoman. I had been counting on Tim to stay with me the night before the parade, help pick up yard signs with his truck, and walk with us in the parade. Instead, he stayed out drinking with his friends. When I spoke with him at one or two in the morning, he said, "I'm with friends, and I can't just leave." At that moment, I realized it wasn't that he couldn't. He didn't want to.

A few days later we talked and I told him it wasn't working out romantically. He didn't seem surprised. I had wanted to remain friends, but that was not what Tim did with ex-girlfriends. I have heard he's married now and really happy, and I'm happy for him.

Did I regret moving to Colorado for this man? Not on your life. I had taken a chance on love and failed spectacularly. I now knew myself as someone who was willing to be that vulnerable. Better yet, a vision for my future also had come alive, and that wouldn't have happened had I not taken the risk of moving across the country.

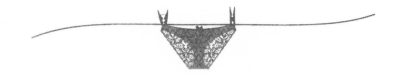

Chapter 10
Mom's Got Cancer

I remember the day like it was yesterday – 2:30pm, August 10th, 2006. I was working from home so I took the call from my Aunt in my office. Mom had gone in for a full hysterectomy, and I was glad to be told that she came out of surgery fine. But nothing could've prepared me for the news I was about to hear.

"Your Mom's hysterectomy went fine," my Aunt said. "They took everything they needed to, but there's something else. Your Mom has cancer. They found it all over the lining behind her uterus." I was stunned. I literally shook my head to get myself present. "What?" I trailed off. My Aunt went on: "Max said not to call. Your Mom is resting and he doesn't want you stressing her out. One of them will call you later."

Again, I shook my head. My vision had blurred, I felt dizzy. "What? How? What? I don't care what Max said, I'm calling Mom. I need to talk to her." My Aunt, in her usual calm way, said: "I wouldn't do that if I were you, sweetie. Max is pretty adamant, but you do what you need to do."

"Okay," I whispered and hung up the phone.

I fell to the floor and curled myself up into a ball and began sobbing. My cats circled me, meowing. Snot ran out of my nose as I sobbed uncontrollably. I looked under the futon couch in my office and pictured my own scared, ashen face looking right back at me as I pressed my backside into the far corner, tucking my five-foot-ten-inch frame into a ball. I could do that and never come out, I thought. Would anyone find me? Would I care? CANCER. My mom has cancer.

I didn't know what to do with myself. A hundred thoughts raced through my mind. I thought about going to see a movie to forget what was happening. Who should I call? What do I do? Do I fly down to Florida? Do I wait to hear? Do I call them? I thought about buying a pack of cigarettes and retreating to the nearest bar to drown myself in a bottle of tequila, but fortunately I had quit both habits cold turkey about seven years before.

Questions flew through my head: What did this mean? How long did Mom have to live? Was she going to die right away? What did the doctors see? Why hadn't they figured this out a long time ago?

Mom had been treated for candida, irritable bowel syndrome and all kinds of other intestinal disorders since the previous spring. When I visited in May, she showed me how swollen her belly was, but that wasn't unusual. There was no cause for alarm. My mom had had intestinal issues as long as I could remember. She was always taking something to go to the bathroom or stop going to the bathroom. I didn't think much of it while I stood in front of her kitchen counter that was covered with all of her homeopathic remedies. After all, this was my mom. She worked out six days a week. She taught tap dancing. She was a vegetarian. She ate only organic fruits and vegetables. She was always reading about the latest in health and nutrition and had always been my health guru. Besides, she was only 66. Her Mom had lived to be 94. There was plenty of evidence to say she would live a long life too.

It wasn't until much later and after doing extensive research that we found out that her symptoms – bloating, abdominal pain, difficulty eating, feeling full quickly after eating and getting nauseated were classic symptoms of Stage I and II Ovarian Cancer. Ovarian Cancer is incredibly hard to diagnose because the early symptoms mimic those most women experience during their monthly menstrual cycle, so they ignore those signs. Most Ovarian Cancer is found by accident after it has metastasized to Stage III and IV. Most patients are diagnosed only after the cancer has already spread to other internal organs, and treatment offers little hope for full remission.

The statistics are staggering. Ovarian Cancer accounts for about three percent of cancers among women, but it causes more deaths than any other cancer of the female reproductive system. A woman's risk of getting ovarian cancer during her lifetime is about 1 in 72. Her lifetime chance of dying from ovarian cancer is about 1 in 100.

I don't know if my mom knew all of this at that time, but she knew at some point because she is the one who corrected me, telling me that she had been diagnosed with Stage IV cancer, not Stage III. When she was diagnosed she had less than an eighteen percent chance of living five years, which meant she was unlikely to see her 71st birthday.

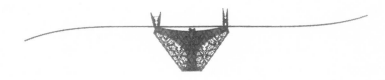

Chapter 11
Just the Facts, Jack

The one thing I did know was that I had to call my mom right away. My hand shakily dialed Mom's cell phone number. I breathed deeply, not wanting my emotional state to rub off on hers. My stepdad answered the phone.

"Max, it's Jennifer," I said through my tears.

"God damn it, I told you not to call your mother. She needs her rest," he responded.

I started sobbing. "I want to hear her voice; I want to know how she is. I had to call." I heard Mom's voice in the background saying to hand her the phone.

"Mamasan?" I said in the smallest voice I'd ever heard come out of my mouth.

"Jeffner," she said into the phone. Jeffner was what my big brother Aaron called me when he was little because he couldn't say Jennifer. That was her pet name for me. I could tell she was pretty drugged up from the pain medication.

"Mommy, I'm sorry, I had to call and hear your voice. I need to know what is going on. Do you need me to come to you right away? What can I do? I have my seminar tonight, but I'll cancel it and come to you," I said.

Mom and I had participated in personal growth and development courses since the early eighties. She wasn't as involved as I was, but we had a common language and a way of speaking to one another that was very truthful, honest and from the heart.

"There is nothing for you to do right now honey. We do not know what the facts are and until we do, there is nothing to do. You go lead your seminar, honey. You go make a difference with the people in your class. That will make you happy. It always does. That will make me happy, too."

I started crying again. I was moved by her incredible strength and generosity, moved by how logical and willing to deal with reality she was. That was the first lesson she taught me: to only deal with the facts and not the stories we were making up based on those facts. We knew what we knew right now, in this moment of time. Anything else was unknown. All of our fears were about what *might* happen, not what was *certain* to happen. So it didn't serve either of us, right now, to ask the bigger questions because we simply didn't have answers. That didn't stop me from having those questions, but Mom didn't want me to preoccupy myself with them. Once again, my mom was consoling me.

"What happened?" I asked. "Well, when the doctor did the hysterectomy she found cancer all around the abdominal wall and in some other areas. An oncological surgeon was operating next door and came in to assist. The doctor removed what she could and in the next few days we will talk to discuss treatment options.

"Mom?" I asked, my voice quavering. "How bad is it? I mean will you...." I couldn't bring myself to ask *that* question. But my mom always knew how to read my mind.

"Honey, we really don't know anything at this point, not until they test the tissue and they stage the cancer. Once they stage it, we'll know how bad it is, and we'll know the treatment options."

"Okay, Mom. You let me know when you want me to come down to see you, okay? I'll call you tomorrow. I love you Mommy, veeerrrry much." My mom responded in kind, with the very long "very." It's what her Mom used to say to us every time we talked, whether by phone or in person, no matter how many times a day. We had continued the tradition throughout the years and most of the time I said it because it was routine. This time it was not.

I took a shower, got dressed but couldn't stop crying. I felt totally helpless. I got in my car and drove to where I was leading my seminar. You know those times you drive somewhere and you have no idea how you got there? I wish that had happened this time. I knew every inch of that journey. It seemed like it took me hours, but it didn't. The drive was exactly as it always had been – same traffic, same highway, same buildings, same trees. Somehow I thought everything should at least look a little different. But it didn't. Everything looked exactly the same, but I knew my life would never be the same again.

I got to the office building and remember sitting at one of the desks, trying to get it together before starting the evening. One of the other leaders walked over to me and gently rested her hand on my shoulder. She was an older, plain looking woman, with soft blue eyes and gray hair. She worked with animals and was internationally known for being a very successful horse whisperer. She simply said: "This is your Mom's journey."

In that moment, I understood what it must feel like for those horses to experience being understood – for some human person to get them, their world, and what it must be like to be them in that moment. I calmed down immediately, my shoulders relaxed; I no longer heard the sound of my own heart beating in my ears. I felt a quiet peace filling my body and realized that it *was* my mom's journey. There was nothing for me to "do" in that moment other than to accept what was going on. I could either resist what was happening and be totally pissed off at the world, or I could accept things just the way they were, and just the way they were not.

Acceptance—not acquiescence—would make all the difference in the world. In acceptance, there was freedom for me to choose how I was going to be in the next moment. In acquiescence, I was left submitting to something, fighting something, or rallying against some enemy—one that I couldn't see. I didn't know how long my mom was going to live. But I knew that feeling sorry for myself or for her was going to make no difference at all. What would make a difference was being fully present with those in the seminar and impacting their lives the way Mom had always impacted mine.

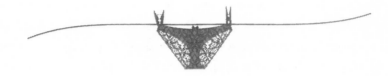

Chapter 12
It's Just Cancer

For the next several months I was on high alert – calling every day to check in to find out if we knew anything new. I spent hours online reading about Ovarian Cancer and alternative therapies. I talked to friends in the healthcare profession and had them refer me to other friends. I talked to energy healers, herbalists, and nutritionists – anyone I could get my hands on and passed all of that information on to Mom and Max. I wanted to be as helpful as I could; after all, my childhood nickname was "Helpful Hannah." (Although to this day I'm not sure that was a compliment, more like a "hey, stop getting in the way," but whatever.)

After a while, Mom's cancer became a part of the routine of life. I lived in Colorado, 2,000 miles away from Sarasota, FL where my mom and Stepdad lived. So, I was not living with my mom's cancer on a daily basis. It wasn't front and center for me all the time. Mom never really seemed sick because she was on the go all the time. She worked out six days a week. She taught tap dancing, and she won awards for her tap performances. In fact, she won "Senior Idol" with her best friend. Mom appeared in plays. She was in a fashion show. She and Max went out to dinner with friends at least four nights a week, and they traveled to see people they knew. These were her retirement years, so she was doing all the things she had been wanting to do and balancing all of that with regular chemo treatments, doctor visits, and Eastern medicine rituals.

So, as time passed I reverted to old habits, namely working a lot and sometimes letting weeks pass without calling. I'd think of calling her but didn't always pick up the phone and dial. Sometimes the time difference prevented me from calling. Sometimes I was in the middle of something and vowed to get to it later, but then it became too late due to the time difference. Inevitably, I'd get a call and hear my mom's voice mocking a stereotypical Jewish New York accent.

"Jennifah—this is your Muthah. It's been three weeks since we tawked. I am cawlling to make you feel guilty. I hope it works. Cawl me baaaa—aaaack." It always worked.

I took it for granted that she would always be on the other end of a phone and that I'd always be able to hear her voice. There is so much I took for granted about our relationship. And the biggest thing was this: we had time. I wanted to believe that, somehow, life didn't have a final curtain call and that there wasn't an endgame. I knew intellectually that we all died, but I couldn't be with it at all. I didn't want to talk about it. I couldn't talk about it.

That Mom would die before my stepdad Max, let alone die at all, simply seemed surreal. I expected Max who was 13 years older to go first.

I had lunch with a dear friend of Mom's a few months after she died. Joanne is an artist who lives near Washington, DC and does textiles and crafts. She and Mom met in Parents without Partners back in the '70s when they both were newly divorced. Joanne told me that Max's age was a big consideration for my mom when deciding to date him. She knew it was predictable that she would end up caring for him, and she took a long, hard look at whether she really wanted to do that. I know she never thought the tables would turn and he'd be the one caring for her.

I was lucky enough to have two sets of parents—my mom and stepdad, and my dad and stepmom. My parents were married to each other for only 13 years, and each had been with their current spouse for over 30 years. I loved them all equally. While my folks' divorce had been hard, I was really happy with the people they had chosen to spend the rest of their lives with. Frankly, I never thought I'd be faced grieving the death of one of my parents without my mom. She seemed immortal to me and I figured she'd be around forever, my grandmother lived to be 94, but Mom died at 71. She was supposed to have at least 23 more years so that, when she died, I'd be an old lady and I'd be ready for it. It was inevitable, but I'd be prepared.

After facing all of this, I'm no longer scared of death because I spent a lot of time reading and researching what happens to us when we die. If you want a terrific book to read, read *Journey of the Soul: A Case Study of Life Between Lives*, because of that book and others I now believe that death isn't the end. I also appreciate the moments I have so much more than before my mom died. Since her death I've tried to live without judgment or worry and to love unconditionally. I'm not a saint by any means. I fail more than I succeed, but each moment is a new opportunity to try again.

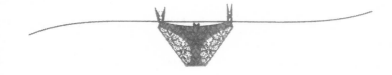

Chapter 13
Are you Kidding Me?

Fast forward to the summer of 2009, I was running for the State House of Representatives in Colorado. I was calling old friends for campaign contributions. Calling and asking for money for my own campaign was the hardest thing I'd ever had to do. I was calling people I hadn't spoken to in years and asking them to donate. I'd say a quick hello followed by, "It's so good to hear your voice. Can I have your money?" Sometimes I was successful, sometimes I was not. I now had so much more compassion for the candidates I used to push to ask for money. No wonder they hated it.

I glanced up from this annoying (but necessary) task to see my husband Adam at the doorway to my office. Something in the way he looked gave me a knot in my stomach. "Did you pay the rent?" I asked. Not one muscle on his face moved as he shook his head slowly from side to side. *Seriously*, I thought? I always had to do everything—work full-time, take care of the house, figure out the childcare schedule with his ex-wife because they don't talk. I asked him to take care of one small thing! "Why not?" I asked with a sneer.

He answered by shrugging his shoulders. I was getting more and more frustrated. "What is it? Are you okay?" He shook his head and took a few steps in to my office, heading toward the futon couch where we had spent hours laughing and giggling together.

Okay this was not him. I stopped being annoyed and focused on him. "What is it honey? Do you not feel good?" He shook his head again. Well if it wasn't physical, what was it? "Is it emotional? Spiritual?" He nodded his head. "Are the kids okay?" I badgered him.

"I can't do this anymore," he said almost silently.

"What do you mean *this*?" I asked.

"Us, I can't be married to you anymore," he responded. My world literally stopped in that moment. I felt like I was in a movie. My eyes went blurry. I walked over to the couch and sat beside him.

"What do you mean you can't be married anymore?" I asked.

"I love you, but I don't love your lifestyle," he said. "*You* have a career." It was his turn to sneer.

Was he kidding me? Had he met me? He knew who he was marrying. He knew my ambition to run for office. In fact, he had told me he totally supported my career and would even move to DC if I we needed to. That was the moment when we were dating – when he sent that email saying he'd move for me – when I gave myself full permission to fall in love with him. And now this? Was he kidding me?

"Are you kidding me?" I asked.

"No, I'm going to pick up the kids and we are not coming back."

He looked at me with no emotion on his face what so ever. I had this weird, out-of-body experience. I started crying, because it felt like that was what I was supposed to do. But honestly, I felt nothing. Was I in shock? Was I numb? Or if I was being honest with myself, had I known this day was coming? I used to sneak out of bed at 2:00am and sit in my office and cry for hours trying not to wake him praying for guidance as to whether I should stay with him or go. I had given my word and wanted to work things out but in those moments our marriage seemed so hard and incredibly devoid of joy.

To make matters worse, Mom's cancer had come back and I was leaving the next day to fly to Florida to be with her. Mom had enjoyed a year of remission but she wanted to have some time with me, so I was flying down for a week. It was also 28 days before the end of the quarter and I had another $5,000 to raise. In that moment while I was crying, snot running down my nose, and my husband about to walk out the door ending the life I knew, all I could think about was how pissed off I was at the inconvenience of the whole thing and how insensitive he was being. Am I that heartless, I thought to myself?

I didn't know what else to say so I pretended like I felt sick to my stomach and ran into the bathroom and shut the door, partially hoping Adam would follow. Instead he chose that moment to escape. I heard the front door slam shut. I burst out of the bathroom and ran after him to confront him at his car.

I was sobbing and begging him to stay. "Where will you go?" I asked. "I don't know," was all he said. But he knew, all right. I later found out he'd been talking to his first wife about getting back together. They'd spent hours on the phone together while he was in a relationship seminar, supposedly working on our marriage. I wondered why he hadn't talked to me about what he was dealing with. Now I knew. He was picking up their kids and moving back in with her—one big, happy family.

Adam was stoic as he got into his car and drove away. There I was, in the middle of my driveway, at the end of a cul-de-sac, in my nice suburban neighborhood, crying, watching my husband's car pull away, and feeling completely helpless and totally alone.

I walked back into the house in a daze. What had just happened? Did he really leave? Was he really not coming back? Did I give a shit? I walked into my office and looked at my phone and the call sheets. I witnessed my own arm extend toward the phone as if to dial another number to ask someone for money, and I stopped mid-reach. What was I doing? Who was I calling? My husband literally just walked out. On some level I hated to admit it to myself, I felt a very real sense of relief. I exhaled slowly letting out a breath I realized I'd been holding in for months.

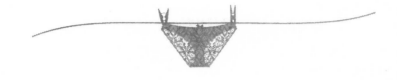

Chapter 14
There, There, It Will Be Okay

When Adam and I got married, I felt like the luckiest woman in the world. I was already past my baby-making prime. In fact, I used to joke that, at the age of 42, I likely had one egg left that was coughed out each month like an old Jewish man hacking up a phlegm ball. I was lucky, though, because not only was I getting a terrific husband who supported me and my dreams, but also he had two wonderful children by his first wife. The two split time with them equally so they already had a Mom. I got the wonderful honor of being a stepmom.

My stepmother, Patricia, had married my dad when I was eleven. Patricia and I were very close. She had an enormous impact on my life. I remember the first time I went with her into New York City where she worked. There she was, this tall, gorgeous, leggy blond in a black leather miniskirt. She turned heads when she walked down the street to her very impressive job at one of the top advertising agencies in the world. She was sophisticated and smart, and she was opinionated without being condescending. She was great with people. She made you feel like you were the only person she was talking to when she was with you. She was both interesting and interested in you.

She had a very creative spirit. It showed in her love of and ingenuity in her cooking. She showed me how to follow the basics of a recipe but then to get inventive. Her creativity showed in the way she dressed, so I encouraged her to take me shopping so I could look as pretty. She encouraged my dad to take me into the city to see a show when I would visit. Now that was the epitome of sophistication for this Midwestern girl—dinner and a show with my dad in the big city. Through her I learned to look at my living space as an artistic expression; I was wowed by the architectural changes she would make to their homes. I took notes on the ways she decorated.

She talked to me like I was a grown up, so I related to her more as a big sister and confidante and not so much as my other mother. I think she wanted it that way. She had always said that she didn't want to interfere or try to take my mom's place. I appreciated that, as did Mom.

I was looking forward to developing that kind of relationship with my own step kids, but first I had to get over my fear of being alone with them.

"They aren't going to break," Adam said to me the first time I was to be alone with them before we got married. "They're kids; they're resilient."

"But what if I do something stupid and accidentally hurt them? Like I leave a burner on and they burn their hand or something?" I replied my eyes wide with fear.

Adam chuckled. "It's called an accident because you didn't mean to do it. If they get burned you put salve on the wound. I'm a nurse, remember," he said. He always had a way of calming me down when I was irrational. It was never in a condescending way, and he'd make me laugh at myself.

Adam had been an ICU nurse for thirteen years, so he had no problem with blood or vomit. I told him early on I couldn't stand the sight of blood and if I had to clean up vomit I'd wind up vomiting, too. He had agreed to take care of any solids or liquids coming out of any orifice of the children's bodies.

He had recently taken a job as a critical care transport nurse, so when he pulled up in the ambulance in front of the house to check on me the first time I was alone with the kids, it made me love him even more. "I told you, you're not going to break them," he'd say with glee in his eyes. "I could break an arm," I'd say being literal. He would just chuckle and shake his head.

I stood in the middle of my office the day he left remembering the loving way Adam had looked at me that day as he got out of the ambulance. Now, twelve thousand thoughts raced through my head. Why hadn't I seen this coming? What were the clues? Sure, we had had our difficulties. We'd been through a lot for a couple who had only been married two years: Mom's cancer; each of us getting new jobs; our moving in together; me figuring out how to be a Stepmom; his son getting ill; and his ex-wife being ill. There were a lot of stressful factors, but I had just figured we would get through it.

Adam wasn't a talker and I had learned early on that if we were going to succeed as a couple, I would always be the one to initiate the hard conversations. I had learned to sit quietly with him and wait for him to talk or gently ask questions and let him know it was okay to say what was on his mind. He always thanked me for it later and each time it became easier and easier. Years after our divorce he acknowledged me for teaching him that it was safe to communicate.

The last time we had spoken was one of the most difficult conversations of our relationship. I was at my wit's end. I was doing my best to arrange our schedules with the kids' Mom so that it could accommodate his work schedule, my travel schedule and give us time alone. But we never got it, Adam always seemed to have something come up, and I was getting more and more resentful and frustrated every week. He'd come home from work, change his clothes and head downstairs to play guitar. I tried to talk to him and find out what was wrong and he repeatedly told me "nothing." I knew it wasn't true but after a while I just gave up. I went about my life doing what I had to do and ignored him and hoped that one day he'd finally talk to me. I knew it wasn't the answer but I was tired from doing all of the work.

That Sunday I was the proverbial teakettle going off after being under intense pressure. I told him that we had to go to marriage counseling because we were so unhappy and nothing was getting any better. "What are they going to do for us?" he asked. It was a good question, one which I didn't have an answer for because I'd never been married before but I figured that an outside viewpoint from a professional could give us the perspective that we needed. I honestly didn't know if I wanted to stay in the marriage but I also knew that I had a history of giving up easily. I wanted a professional opinion that I could trust.

I had been working on myself throughout our marriage and for a few years Adam and I had participated in personal growth and development seminars together and used the tools for communicating all of the time. We had a good marriage, until we didn't. I realized that around the time he stopped going, because his new job was so intense, was the time things between us started really breaking down. I couldn't save our marriage on my own so maybe, I figured, working together would be less scary for him and be a great way for us to grow as a team?

"Are you willing to work on the marriage?" I asked. He nodded his head. "Well if you won't go to marriage counseling, maybe therapy would be a good idea?" I offered. "They are just going to tell me I don't know how to communicate," he said with his lip curled. We talked a bit more and he finally agreed to take another seminar – but not with me, which was okay. He signed up for the "Relationship Seminar" – perfect I thought. He can come home and share with me what he is learning and I can share with him and we will cause a breakthrough and get through this! He started in June, and by July, I had a new husband.

He was affectionate, kind, and complimentary, and we had finally worked out the childcare schedule with his ex-wife, leaving me with alone time and us with romantic time. I was happy and peaceful for the first time in months and he seemed to be so too. I thought things were getting better. How wrong I was! What kind of person was I married to that could have played it so cool, pretending everything was okay while plotting to move out? What kind of person was I that I was so incredibly blind and so incredibly stupid? How could I have missed all of this?

The only person I wanted to talk to at that moment was my mom. Maybe she could make sense of it all. "Hi Max, it's me, can you get Mom on the phone, too?" I asked. I started crying.

"Sure Jen, what's wrong?" he asked. "You okay?" I asked him again to just get Mom on; I couldn't bear telling this tale twice. "Will do. Hold on." My mom got on the phone and I told them both what happened.

"So, when you pick me up tomorrow, I don't know how I'll be," I said. "I just wanted to give you a warning before I get there."

They reassured me as best as they could. The last thing Mom needed was for me to be a mess but that small child in me really wanted her to do that: to take me into her arms like she used to and smooth my hair and say, "There, there. Shhh. Shhh. It will be okay."

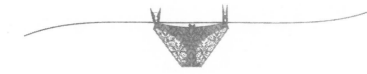

Chapter 15
What Will People Say?

hung up the phone and sat down on the futon having no idea what to do next. Who to call? Who to tell? Who not to tell? What do I say, exactly? How do I say what there is to say? Maybe I shouldn't say anything. Some childish belief in me thought that if I didn't tell a soul— if I didn't say a word—then it wouldn't be real; it couldn't be real. I was numb. I was stunned. I was frozen in time. Low guttural sounds began forming in my throat and I choked out a sob.

I knew I didn't want to be alone so I picked up the phone and made a call to one of my closest girlfriends, Ellen. I told her everything that had happened, repeating some of it because I was crying so hard. She invited me to her home, but she lived an hour-and-a-half away. I still had to pack and didn't trust myself on the road; my entire body was shaking uncontrollably. I was still numb trying to process it all.

Unfortunately, none of my very close girlfriends lived nearby, or they had families of their own so couldn't really just pick up and come over. I had become one of those women I didn't like, the one who, after she found boyfriend or got married, stopped seeing her friends on a regular basis. More than that, I didn't know what I wanted to hear. Did I want consoling? Or would that make me cry harder and go deeper into my well of despair? Did I want tough love—someone to tell me to snap out of it, that I deserved better and to get on with my life? How did I get on with my life when this news was merely hours old?

I wasn't sure what I needed right then. But I did have a campaign to run, and this was incredibly inconvenient and could very likely impact my public image. People would talk. They would say things. I had to control what got out there if anyone found out. I had a job to do and people's investment to protect.

Oh G-d, I hated myself. This was exactly what Adam was talking about. I had a career – had ambitions come to mean more to me than our family? Why was I thinking about how this would impact the campaign? Shouldn't I be thinking about the kids and how this would impact them? In that moment, I made it all okay by telling myself I was being practical. It will impact my mood and my ability to get things done so my campaign manager needed to know. I took a deep breath, picked up the phone and dialed him.

He dropped everything and came over. Here is this kid in his twenties consoling a forty-something woman whose husband had just left her. He didn't know what to do, so he just held my hand as I cried. I think he made me some food or at least offered to. I don't even remember what we spoke about. I just remember him sitting across from me handing me Kleenex, and saying over and over, "That sucks. That so sucks. That's such bullshit. That sucks." It did suck and at that moment that is exactly what I needed to hear.

Somehow I packed my suitcase that night. I think I slept but don't remember exactly when I fell asleep, because the last thing I remember is simply crying and crying. I was feeling so sorry for myself, sorry for Adam and me, sorry about whatever I had done, sorry that I had ever entertained the thought of ending things. I started going over every moment of our three years together in my head; dissecting each interaction with Adam or the kids or his ex-wife. I thought about every time I had a short fuse, every time I did something really mean, every time something went wrong. If there was even a small chance it was my fault, I found that memory and cried about my actions. It wasn't a pleasant thing to do, but I couldn't help it. My mind had a mind of its own.

I went to the airport in a daze. My face was puffy. I walked with my eyes cast downward. I didn't want people to see my face. I didn't want them to look into my eyes, see the devastation, and give me one of those, "Ah, poor baby," looks. I don't think I could've taken an ounce of compassion because it would've only added to my sorrow and misery. I attempted to detach myself from everyone around me. But it seemed like everywhere I looked, people were staring at me. The more they stared, the more I cried. I couldn't help it. I attempted to make myself small. It was a time when I wished I was five-foot-two so I could blend in, instead of five-foot-ten.

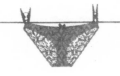

Chapter 16
Make it Work

I checked in at the gate, and my phone rang. It was Ellen.

"How are you?" she asked.

She knew the answer, but she also knew I'd want her to ask the question. Outside of my folks and my campaign manager, she was the only one I had told in my close circle. We both led seminars and being on that team meant that we kept nothing about our personal lives hidden. We knew everything about each other. We were committed to each other's happiness. We knew that when we stood together for the possibility of something, there was very little that could get in our way.

"I'm okay," I didn't have to say much more. Ellen knew I wasn't "okay" in any way, shape or form, but I was okay for now.

I was okay in this moment. I wasn't dying. I was getting through the day.

"What do you want Jen?" she asked. "I want to send something out to our team so that they know your intention and can get behind you." I swallowed hard. I didn't know. I only knew the extreme heartache I was feeling right in that moment as I thought about a future of never seeing Adam or the kids again.

"I think I'm crazy but I want this marriage to work. I'm intending that we stay together, and that we work things out. That whatever we are up against, we get in communication and sort it out."

Ellen choked back her own sobs. Ellen had done one of the blessings at our wedding. Adam and Ellen's husband had bonded over their love of cycling. Our kids had played together. She and her family had been friends with us and were one of the few couples that we had done things with. She asked me who to send it to—our team in Denver and our leadership team from across the West Coast region? "Yes. Send it to Susan Freele, too," I said through my tears.

You have to picture Susan. She grew up in Philadelphia and had the attitude of a New Jersey mobster, she was sweet and kind but really protective of the people she loved. Susan had been my confidante back in 2008 when I was being intensively trained as a coach. She had stood beside me while I went through the eye of the needle. She had coached me through some very delicate times in my marriage. I knew she wanted me to be happy. She weighed nearly three hundred pounds and was about five-foot-two. At this point she had lost a hundred pounds, but her personality was still as big as her body used to be.

"I will Jen," Ellen said. "You have a safe flight. I love you."

"I love you, too."

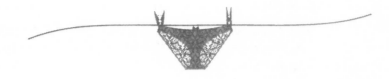

Chapter 17
Moms Are Like Gods

spent the week with Mom and Max. I had been looking forward
to running on the beach, to enjoying the sunsets, to enjoying the
warmth and moisture of the Florida air, to being fully with my mom,
and to being fully available to her and Max. I had plans to go to chemo
with the two of them, to tap class with Mom, and to see some of her
other friends I had gotten acquainted with. Every evening at five o'clock,
the neighbors would gather by the pool, enjoy a cocktail and snacks, and
laugh and laugh. I was looking forward to all of that.

But now the sun pissed me off. People being cheerful pissed me
off. The wild peacocks pissed me off. The fruit trees pissed me off. The
swimming pools pissed me off. I had always muscled through situations

because I found a way to rise above and keep going. People admired me for that—my tenacity, my resilience. Now I couldn't muster those character traits if I tried. I was miserable and crying most of the time. I went to sleep crying. I woke up, and there was bliss for a few brief seconds. Then, BOOM, reality set in and I would start to cry. Mom bought me a homeopathic remedy called "nerve tonic" and I popped those little herbal pills like candy. It helped, but nothing could make reality disappear.

Mom generally wasn't ready to have company until nine or nine-thirty in the morning. She was tired from the cancer and the chemo. Things simply took her longer than usual. I knew to give her some time in the morning.

It took everything I had to get out of bed that first morning after I arrived. My legs felt like lead. I was hungry but didn't feel like eating. I wanted coffee but couldn't bring my hands to go through the motions. I just wanted my mommy to take care of me. I felt so helpless and so darned alone. The one person I used to talk to about everything was, at that moment, the one person who was the source of my suffering: Adam.

I picked up the phone and called Mom but there was no answer. I tried the house phone and got the answering machine. Well, at least Max was gone so I could have time alone with Mom. Likely, she was in the bathroom. It was already nine-thirty, so I decided to get dressed and walk over to their apartment. She should be up.

I walked outside and the smell of the morning hit my nostrils—all grapefruit and fresh earth. The glint of the sun bouncing off the leaves blinded me as I put on my sunglasses. Tears started rolling down my face. I wished Adam and the kids had had a chance to be here. The kids would have loved this place, I thought, as I slowly walked over to Mom's. I wasn't moving fast. I couldn't move fast. I felt like I had one of those lead mats thrown over my body, the ones they use to protect your vital organs when you get an x-ray. Everything felt heavy. Just then I stepped on a small branch and nearly twisted my ankle. God, I was so pathetic. I started crying harder, hoping no one would see me. I wished I could disappear.

I arrived at Mom's door, only to find it shut. Uh oh. Maybe today was a bad day. Maybe she needed extra time. Maybe I should go back, so I turned around to go, and then stopped. I took a deep breath and let out a whimper. I turned back around and brought my hand up to the door and froze. I didn't want to knock, but I needed one of her hugs. I didn't want to bother her. I shouldn't bother her. I put my arm back down next to my body. I felt so helpless, as if deciding to knock on that door was the hardest decision I would ever have to make in my entire adult life. So I just stood there, frozen, hand raised. Finally, I knocked on the door and waited. I knocked again and waited. I started crying silently. I started keening, making that low moaning sound you hear from hurt animals. It was a guttural sound, unlike any noise that had ever come out of my mouth. I waited a few more moments. Then, I turned around and slowly walked back to where I was staying.

As I arrived at the apartment, my phone rang and it was Mom sounding so cheerful, just like she always did. "Hi honey, I was in the back bathroom, but I forgot to open the door. I'm so sorry, come back over," she said.

I burst into tears from all the frustration and exhaustion. In the dreams I had the night before, things were okay. Then I woke up to the sharp reality that my husband had walked out. All of that emotion ran out of my mouth and nose. "I don't think I can Mom. I don't think I have it in me to walk back over." I stuttered nearly inaudibly. I was so tired.

"Do you want me to come over there?" she asked. I didn't know. I honestly didn't know. I didn't want her to have to get dressed and come over. I knew she would never leave the house without her wig and makeup. If she wasn't already dressed I didn't want to make her get dressed. But I wanted her to come over, too.

"I don't know, Mom. I don't know what I want—to walk over there? It was so hard earlier to just put one foot in front of the other. I don't know if you should come here because if you are tired and want to hang out, you should take time to do that." I started crying even harder. "I don't know what I want to do."

"Ah, honey, I'll be right over. You just stay there," she said. She came over and took me into her arms, smoothed my hair and said, "There, there. It will be all right. Mommy's here," just like she did when I was little girl. I sighed and melted into her embrace, and for one very brief moment, I believed her words to be true. I believed her just like I did when I was a little girl when Moms were like G-ds, and everything they said usually came true.

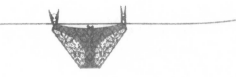

Chapter 18
Men are Like SEPTAs

I spent that week in Florida trying to make sense of it all in between my bouts of crying and sleepless nights. I talked to Adam a few times. It became very clear to me that his mind was made up. I suppose I should've known that from the apartment searches and the emails I had discovered. Whatever conversations we could have had or should have had, there was no turning back for him now. I didn't know what I had done to make him give up and leave but he couldn't answer. All he said was: "I don't hate you," but I didn't believe him. His actions spoke louder than his words.

I wondered a lot about what I could have done differently. I spent those sleepless hours going over every argument we had, every time I yelled at the kids, and all the times I over-reacted. I wondered if any one of those things had not happened, would things be different than they were today? I couldn't answer that. Adam wouldn't tell me. The bottom line was he was barely speaking to me.

I was still astonished that he had gone back to his first wife. This was the same woman he had ranted about. This was the same woman who had begged me to intervene between the two of them and work out their childcare schedule when neither was speaking to the other. I had stood for both of them to get along. I had stood for us to be one big happy family. Now *they* were the big happy family, and I was the odd person out.

One morning my mom took me to talk with her spiritual advisor, Reverend Duffy. Duffy, as she was known to her friends, ran the Center for Spiritual Living. The Center was based on the teachings of the founder, Ernest Holmes, who believed that there was no separation between man and God, or Christ Consciousness, as Duffy called it. The first time I went to the Center with my mom, hearing the Christ reference made me uncomfortable because I'd been raised Jewish. I talked to Duffy about it.

"Just ignore the Christ reference, Jen," Duffy told me. "You can substitute whatever you want—G-d, Buddha, Yahweh, the Light, Mother Mary—whatever higher power you believe in. Fact is humanity lives in this fallacy that we are separated from what I call 'Godsource', and we are not. We are one, and that's all I'm saying." I fell in love with Duffy in that moment. From then on, her presence always calmed me down. She was part therapist, part minister, part Mom and a total and complete space of unconditional love.

I told Duffy what had happened and what Adam and I had been dealing with over the three years of our relationship. I shared all of my heartache, my anger toward Adam and his ex-wife, and, finally, my anger at myself. I really was trying to find *the* reason Adam left. If only I had *that* key.

"I used to yell at the kids. Adam told me that Shawn was glad we were getting divorced because I was mean," I said, crying.

"Ah, Jen," Duffy said. "A lot of kids think parents are mean when they are disciplining them."

I knew what Duffy meant. Shawn had said the same thing to me about his own Mom when Adam and I got married. I had been the nice Mom and she had been the mean one. Truth be told, I liked that I was the nice one at the time; I was the savior. I didn't tell the kids that. I told them that she was doing the best she could, but I certainly gloated over what he'd said. Boy, karma is a bitch.

I don't remember everything Duffy and I talked about, but I do recall feeling relieved. At the end of our few hours together, I had accepted what was going on. However, that didn't mean I was giving up on our marriage or was giving in. I didn't like or want what was happening; yet the facts were the facts. Adam had left. He wanted to move everything out. He was staying with his ex-wife. That seemed pretty final but who really knew what the future held. I called Adam and told him I accepted his decision. I even told him what furniture to take because I didn't want him moving into his own apartment without any furniture or beds for the kids.

I wasn't giving up, or giving in, but I was accepting the fact that Adam had moved out and that he was unhappy. God knows we were both unhappy. I remember a time when Adam was on his computer and I was sitting on the couch in the family room, crying and saying, "I just want us to be happy." Adam said he wanted that too, but I never thought splitting up was going to be the answer. Like I said I'd thought about splitting up, too—more than I'd care to admit—at different points. But I would never really have left. I loved him too much.

On the way back to Denver, my "New Jersey Mobster" Susan called me. I knew she would.

"Jennifer, its Susan. I saw your email and after I saw it I called Ellen within 10 minutes, but I wasn't able to call you until now. What the heck is going on?" she asked.

I gave her the shorthand version. I told her about spending the afternoon with Duffy and how I had come to peace with things afterward.

"Jennifer, look," Susan began to lecture. "I'm going to tell you something my mother told me. My mother said a lot of stuff to me growing up that was completely useless. But she said this one thing that made a helluva lot of sense."

I smiled to myself. Only Susan could talk that way about her Mom. She loved her Mom. I knew that because I had heard the stories. Susan just didn't mince words.

"Jennifer, men are like SEPTAs. You know what SEPTA is?" she asked.

"No Susan, what is SEPTA?" I responded.

"Southeastern Pennsylvania Transit Authority. It's a subway train. My mother used to say, men are like SEPTAs. When you wait on the platform another one will come along in twenty minutes."

It was the first time I had laughed in three days, and it felt really, really good. Leave it to Susan.

"I'm not saying you shouldn't stand for your marriage and make it work. But remember there will always be another man to come along," she said. "Is there anything you need?"

I told her that the best thing was that she had made me laugh. I told her to keep my intention to stay with my husband in her prayers, whomever she prayed to, and we hung up the phone. I couldn't wait to tell Mom what she had said.

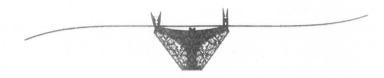

Chapter 19
I'm Definitely Not O.K.

My stepfather Max convinced me to get a lawyer.

He'd been protective of me since the day we met. I was home one weekend from college and my boyfriend and I were out riding on his motorcycle. Neither one of us was wearing a helmet since there was no helmet law in Ohio at the time. Max came roaring off the porch when we pulled up and yelled at us both. I was nineteen and was really pissed off at this dude who thought he was my dad but wasn't. He was embarrassing me in front of my boyfriend in front of my house in broad daylight where the neighbors could hear. I couldn't understand that that was his way of showing me his love at the time, though I did realize it many years later.

Max had wanted me to get a lawyer because he didn't want Adam to have any kind of an advantage over me because he had been divorced before. Max wanted me with someone who knew the system and knew what they were doing. I called my dear friend Robert, but it turned out that he couldn't represent me because we had hired him to represent Adam during a legal matter with his first wife. Robert referred me to someone else and I set up an appointment. I wasn't certain if the outcome was going to be an actual divorce, but Max convinced me to set up the appointment to talk things through.

"I know you may not feel like this is a good idea right now, Jen, but your Mom and I do." He smiled his little smile at me, and that was his kind of hug of encouragement. I took a deep breath. Now it was time to tell Adam.

I called Adam and told him I had accepted his decision. Then I told him I was hiring a lawyer.

"Why they hell are you hiring a lawyer if you are okay with getting a divorce?" he exploded at me over the phone.

"Okay with getting a divorce? I never ever said I was okay with it. I said I accepted it. I accepted it because what else am I to do but accept what is happening right now? I'm not okay with it. I don't agree with it. I think it sucks." I screamed at him. "What other choice do I have?"

In that moment I was glad he was gone. I was glad he had gotten the hell out of the house. In that moment I never wanted to see him again. I told him that he could hire whomever he wanted. I told him to pack all of his and the kids' stuff and get it out of the house by the time I got back. Then I slammed down the phone.

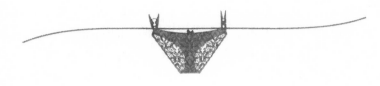

Chapter 20
What Happened?

The week with Mom and Max was therapeutic, but now I was facing going back to the home I had created with Adam and the kids. This was the place where I had picked out the kid's bedspreads and sheets so they could feel at home, safe and comfortable in this new place with Daddy's new wife. It was where we had entertained friends, and I had cooked family meals as we gathered around the dining room table. It was the home with our little fish tank and the beta fish I had bought as a surprise for the kids but became attached to as my own.

I was about to enter into a place that was decorated with wedding gifts and had tiny handprints on the walls from the kids. It was full of memories of my dream marriage. Now at least half the house would be completely devoid of furniture. Adam had emptied the downstairs.

We lived in a four-bedroom, two-bath house. Our bedroom, the living room, dining room, kitchen, and the room that doubled as my office and our TV room were upstairs. The downstairs had the family room, the kids' bedrooms, their bathroom, and an area where they could play and watch their shows. I told Adam to take everything from the downstairs with him. The kids' beds and bedroom furniture had come from their old house so, of course, that was going. The leather living room set I had gotten for free off some college kids on Craigslist and Adam's office/man-cave furniture went with him, too.

I called my good friend Becky and asked if she could come over and just be with me as I entered the house. I sat in my driveway crying until she got there. I didn't know what it would feel like. Adam had told me he hadn't gotten everything and would be coming back a few more times. He had made it sound like the entire move was an emergency evacuation. He had thrown as much as he could into the back of his car and U-Haul and got out as quickly as he could. I didn't know what demons were chasing him, but I knew without a doubt they had my face and name attached to them.

Becky arrived and I shakily took her hand as we entered the house. There was an eerie quiet and a blanket of sadness draped over the house. The sun was shining outside but none of those rays seemed to penetrate. I opened up windows and doors to get fresh air. I put my suitcase in the bedroom and sighed deeply as I saw the empty closets and drawers.

"Ready to go downstairs?" Becky asked me.

"Sure."

She took my hand as best she could as we navigated our way downstairs. I had imagined what it would look like, and I was pretty much dead on. Still, the reality of the situation smacked me upside the head like a whiffle bat hitting the side of a garage. THWACK.

It wasn't just that the furniture was gone and the kids' rooms were empty. The place looked dirty, desperate, sad and lonely. It was devoid of any tiny reminder that people had lived in these rooms, that laughter had rung out, or that Christmas presents had been unwrapped. It was a barren wasteland, and I could barely be with it.

"Come on, let's go upstairs," Becky said.

I silently followed her up the stairs. We sat at the kitchen table.

"What happened?" she asked finally.

Becky was a close friend. We had known each other fifteen years. She had hosted a barbecue for my out of town family and guests the day before Adam and I got married. She always hosted my annual birthday party. She was someone I could tell everything to, someone who wouldn't bullshit me. I knew she wouldn't try to solve my problems, or tell me things would be okay. She'd listen and, when the time was right, she'd hold me to account for my part in the failure of the marriage. She knew that now was not that time. She just wanted to know what had happened.

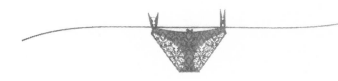

Chapter 21

At Least I'm Not as Bad as the Guests on Jerry Springer

The next three months passed in a blur. I still had my full-time job. I was still running for office. I was traveling for work. I was in meetings for my campaign. I was calling and meeting with voters. I was meeting with unions to get endorsements. I was out every evening. I was raising money. No one but those closest to me knew what my life was really like.

Wake up. Pause for a moment to catch my breath and realize the reality of the situation. Call someone. Not just anyone. I had a handful of very close friends on speed dial.

"Hi, it's me," I'd say.

"How are you?" they would ask.

"I'm okay. I don't feel like doing anything," I'd respond.

They would listen without saying a word, and then we'd proceed to figure out what my next steps were, literally. How did I put one foot in front of the other? Sometimes they would tell me to go out for a walk or go into my garden, knowing full well how much being in nature soothed my soul. Sometimes they would tell me to eat because I had forgotten to or didn't feel like it. Sometimes they would tell me to take a shower. More often than not, when I was done with one task I would call them back and ask what to do next. Day after day, this happened.

I remember one day vividly. I was at my home computer working. My company had been extremely generous in allowing me to work from home knowing the full story about what had recently happened. There I was, trying to respond to emails, trying to edit a document, trying to read news articles, and trying to stop crying. I willed myself to stop. I couldn't stop. I got up and walked around and couldn't stop. I couldn't focus. I called my friend Barry.

"You okay, hon?" He asked.

"Noooooo," I wailed. "I can't stop crying. I can't concentrate. I can't do anything today. I'm so sad. I'm so very sad. It hurts, Barry. It hurts so much. Make it stop. When will it ever stop?"

Barry was silent on the other end of the phone, absorbing my words. I knew he didn't have the answer, nor did I expect him to. I just needed to say what was going on in my head so I could get the thoughts to stop bouncing around like a freaking fly trapped under a glass.

"What do you feel like doing?" he quietly asked me.

I stopped. What did I feel like doing? I had no idea. I mostly was obsessed by what I didn't want to do and what I didn't feel like doing, which was most of my life right then and there. But his question made me stop and think.

"I guess if I could do anything, I'd sit on the couch wrapped in a blanket, bawl my eyes out, and watch a Jerry Springer episode so I could see how much more messed up other people's lives are than my own," I said giggling through my tears.

"That is a great idea!" he shouted gleefully over the phone. "I think you should do that. Sit on the couch, cry and watch Jerry Springer, then call me back."

So I did. I sat on the couch and watched Jerry Springer for about thirty minutes and simply bawled. I wailed. I screamed. I pounded my fists on the couch. I flung myself onto that couch and tossed and turned like a four year-old who was just denied her box of fruity tic-tac's in the middle of a grocery store aisle, certain that one "no" was the end of the world. I gave up resisting that I should be doing anything else or being any other way but sad and crying. I let it all go. It was a beautiful, deep, soul-cleansing cry. When I was done, I was done. I breathed deeply. I walked outside to enjoy the sunshine and I felt refreshed. I called Barry to tell him I was okay and to thank him for being there for me.

"You bet hon," he said.

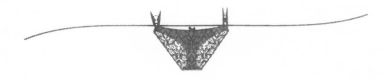

Chapter 22
The Woman in the Mirror

I talked to my mom daily but I tried not to talk about her cancer unless she brought it up. She and Max were guiding me through the divorce process to make sure I was taken care of – Mom always put others before herself. That's what Mom's do, right?

While Adam said he didn't hate me, I didn't believe him. He looked at me with contempt and disgust every time he had to come to the house to pick up more stuff. He wore his hatred of me like a huge splash of paint that was flung on a giant canvas, dripping slowly toward the bottom, covering every inch of cotton. I tried to get an answer, to figure out what I did to deserve this kind of treatment, to find some logical explanation for it all. The only thing he said is that he felt I had lied to him. He thought I had told him that I would be willing to quit my job and stay at home and take care of him and kids. Seriously?

Everyone who ever knew me knew how important my career was to me and how important it was to me to follow my dream of running for office. I thought he did too. I remember when we first started dating he sent me an email letting me know he done a lot of thinking and that even though his kids were in Colorado and cycling was in Colorado, if my career took me back to Washington DC, he would come with me. When I got that email I felt like for the first time in my life my partner got me and supported me. That was my signal that it was safe to fall in love. I thought he was entirely supportive of my career, just as I was supportive of his. I didn't know how our communication had gotten so twisted.

At some point I realized I would never get the answer I wanted to hear. Nothing he could say would satisfy my deep desire to understand *why*. I really only wanted him to drop to his knees and beg for forgiveness for what he done. But that would absolve me of any responsibility and I had been there, too. It was now up to me to take a good hard look at myself. Truth be told, I didn't want to. I wanted to blame him. I wanted to blame his ex-wife. I wanted to blame all of the circumstances.

On the campaign trail, constituents would ask me all kinds of questions about the issues. Most of them centered on public education, but they also included everything from my stance on gay marriage and abortion to the environment and stoplights at intersections. Inevitably I would close with these words: "You will always know where you stand with me. I have a deep-seated conviction to tell the truth and act with integrity because, at the end of the day, I'm the one who has to go to sleep with myself and wake up and look at my own face in the mirror each morning. Mine is the only face I'll ever see."

Well it was time for me to take a good, long, hard look in the mirror. It wasn't about finding blame or feeling at fault – that leaves me as a victim. It was about whether I was willing to be cause in the matter of my life; cause in the matter as in responsible for how my life was going – the good, the bad and the ugly? Was I wiling to play the hand I was dealt? If I wasn't, then I'm a victim of the card game. If I am willing to be responsible, then I could look at the circumstances of my life and ask myself "What am I supposed to learn here?" or "What did I do that didn't align with my values?" or "What did I step over or turn a blind eye to?" I could either continue to be a victim or face the facts. As I thought about this, the first event that came to mind had happened the previous March.

The kids had come to live with us full-time because their Mom was going through some really tough times. Adam and I had never discussed how that would work, in reality. We both had full-time jobs. I traveled a week or more a month. Adam often worked nights and weekends because he was the newest guy on the job. This also was the time that I was gearing up to announce my decision to run for the statehouse. The mistake I made was never speaking to Adam about whether I should run or not, given our new situation.

I didn't talk it through with my husband because, at some level, I rationalized that I already had his approval. The truth is I didn't want him to tell me no. Instead, I consulted my career advisor, confidant and best friend who told me: "This is a time when the kids need to see an adult follow their dreams." I made that make sense to me. After all, why would I let all of the groundwork I had laid go to waste? I went home and told Adam I was running. I didn't ask for his opinion. I didn't explain my thinking. I didn't ask him to sort it out with me to figure out how to have it all work – for both of us. I just told him how it was going to be and expected him to fall in line.

Did this one action cause our marriage to fall apart? Doubtful. But I could be responsible for operating independently instead of as a team – which is how we always did things previously. It definitely left me distant from Adam in a way I hadn't experienced previously and I'm sure it left him feeling like he didn't matter. When we spoke about this a few years later he said that situation hadn't impacted him and honestly that didn't matter. What mattered was my ability to see where I had become distant; where I had stopped creating team; where I had checked out of the marriage.

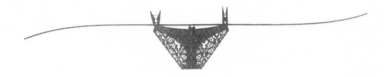

Chapter 23
Happy Seventieth Birthday

It was December 23, 2009, and my mom was turning seventy.

Mom officially had had cancer for three years and four months. From the moment she was diagnosed at age sixty-six, we had been planning her seventieth birthday party. Initially, it was a way to get her mind—and mine—off what she was dealing with in those early months of uncertainty. Then, in her typical fashion, Mom did a lot of research on the Internet and found out that statistically she had less than an eighteen percent chance of living five more years. "Why can't I be part of that eighteen percent?" she asked. No reason at all, I thought. "You are right Mom" I told her. "We are going to plan your seventieth birthday party and when you reach that, we're going to plan your seventy-fifth." I took comfort in envisioning her surrounded with friends, celebrating her life, cutting her cake, and listening to the speeches that would be given. It was much more uplifting then dwelling on, "What if she doesn't make it?"

I knew how important it was to envision a cancer-free future, whether I believed it 100% or not. Many years earlier a friend's fifteen-year-old daughter had been diagnosed with acute myeloid leukemia, a cancer that starts inside the bone marrow. It is rarely found in people under forty and is more common in men than women. Hers was an extremely unusual case. At the time she was diagnosed, the prognosis was very grim. To undergo treatment, she had to live in the intensive care unit of the hospital for forty-five days. These long periods of treatment had to be repeated many times.

What her family found was that when her white blood cell count was elevated—a sign that the cancer was raging through her body—they would encourage her to talk. About what? Anything and everything: how afraid she was, how mad she was, how unfair things were, how much she hurt, how much she hated being in the hospital for so long, and how much she loved her parents and her family and friends. What they found, again and again, was after she said it all, her white blood cell counts would go down and she would start feeling better.

I guess it was a lesson I was storing away for use with my mom. In fact, many of the talks we had had during her cancer years consisted of me simply asking Mom what was on her mind, then waiting patiently for her response. Sometimes that took a while but by the end of every conversation, she felt lighter and happier.

Creating Mom's birthday party gave us a placeholder for the future, I figured. As the weeks turned into months and the months turned into years, I had actually forgotten about that conversation, but apparently my mom had not.

When I arrived in Florida three days before her birthday, Max pulled me aside to tell me that her tap students had planned a surprise luncheon for her the next day. Oh great, I thought, she *hates* surprises. My grandmother used to give her a surprise party every year for her birthday and I remember her telling me how much she hated it. I didn't really get why because I would've loved a surprise party. But Mom liked being in control and knowing what was around the next corner.

I knew her well enough, however, to know that she would be delighted with the surprise no matter what. She never let on otherwise. All of us, elegantly dressed, sat at a long table in a friend's home with fine china and gorgeous food, surrounded by friends from tap class and book club. The tap class had chipped in and bought Mom a scarf made from the most delicate gossamer wool fabric, perfect for her since she was always cold. The color was a deep rose that brought color to Mom's cheeks. She draped it dramatically over one shoulder and looked ecstatic. Pictures were taken and many kind words expressed.

As Mom and I sat next to each other on a bench, she turned to me with tears in her eyes.

"Do you remember when we planned my seventieth birthday party?" she asked me.

It took me a moment to remember, and then I looked at her with wide eyes.

"Remember we said that I'd be celebrating my seventieth birthday? And here we are," she said taking my hand.

As much of a performer as my mom was, she also was a very private person. She didn't like to show emotion in front of others. Her cancer had increased that behavior. She always said that she felt great. When she wasn't feeling up to doing something, she simply didn't go out.

"Nobody here realizes how significant this is," she said to me. "Unless, of course, you told them. Did you?" she asked. "Is that why they planned the party?"

"I didn't say a word. They have no idea."

"Well this makes it truly a special day then, doesn't it? I wasn't sure I would make it this far," she said, squeezing my hand.

I stopped breathing for a moment. My mom had those thoughts? Whew. Of course she did. I remembered back to my friend's daughter again. The night she turned sixteen, I was staying with her and made her stay up past midnight to celebrate. When the clock struck twelve, we high-fived each other, and she burst into tears. "I didn't think I'd make it," she said crying. I started crying too because I had those same thoughts but didn't want to say them. So, of course Mom was no different.

I couldn't have thrown a better 70th birthday for Mom if I had planned it myself. As I sat next to her and looked around the table I got goosebumps. For some unknown reason I had the sense that she'd never see her 75th birthday.

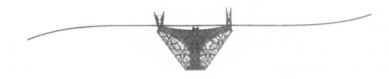

Chapter 24
Should I Stay or Should I Go Now?

*A*fter I returned to Colorado, life went on as usual for the next year or so. Mom continued to teach tap. We had our weekly calls (or semi-weekly as the case may be). I was still traveling a lot but arranged to get down to Florida as often as I could. She continued with her chemotherapy regime, weekly visits with her doctors and specialists, and cheery updates to family and friends. Maybe she was right. Maybe she would be one of those eighteen percent. Life seemed oddly normal for the first time in a long time.

But on February 3, 2011, our world changed once again. Mom had gotten out of the hospital at the end of January; her cancer had spread to her intestines making it difficult for her to keep food down or eliminate waste from her body. She had been in the hospital for over a week while they watched her to see if she would need surgery to remove the blockage. But Mom had other ideas. No surgery. She had willed herself to eat, keep the food down, and start eliminating waste so that she could be discharged from the hospital. Her surgeon allowed it but assured her he would be seeing her in a few weeks.

He told her that it was only a matter of time until the tumors grew back and blocked her intestines once again. He further explained that once the cancer invaded her intestines and her body stopped eliminating waste properly, there wasn't much more that they could do. Surgery was an option, but it was unclear whether it would make any difference or not. The surgeon could not know the degree of the blockage until he had opened up my mother's stomach.

I often told her that I would come at any time, that I would and could figure out a way to work remotely, but she always declined. "I'm fine!" she'd say brightly. I never knew if she was in denial or whether she felt that my coming would be an admission of the beginning of the end. From the beginning, Mom maintained an upbeat positive attitude, often consoling me. But this time when we spoke on the phone something was very different. She didn't sound as certain and confident as before. She sounded beaten down, defeated, and exhausted. Was she admitting that cancer had won?

I put my head down on the desk in front of me and wept. I thought about everything that was already going on in my life for the month: conferences, speeches, and classes I was teaching. I felt stupid that I was thinking about these mundane things. I felt drained and discouraged. I was mad at myself because, damn it, it was my turn to be strong. I felt so helpless and alone. I remember repeating to myself, "I don't know what to do. I don't know what to do." I knew I could call any one of my friends, but I didn't know what to say to them, and I didn't know what I wanted to hear.

The phone rang, and it was my colleague Frank. He and I had become close friends over the years. I had stood by him when he went through a very difficult family situation years before. He had come to me before a meeting with tears in his eyes. "My wife left me yesterday," he said. "I don't know how coherent I'll be today." I just looked into his eyes with as much compassion as I could muster and put my hand on his arm. "I'm so sorry. You don't have to say a word, and if you need to leave, just say so." Something about that moment bonded the two of us and we went from just being colleagues to becoming friends as we both went through divorce, he figured out how to be a single Dad to four boys, and I figured out how to deal with my mom's cancer.

As soon as I saw who it was, I picked up the phone and started sobbing. I told him everything all in a rush: how scared I was of losing my mom; how it wasn't fair; how I wished I could figure out if this was the right time to go to her; how I had so much going on that month and couldn't do it all; and how I didn't know what to do. How I wasn't ready. Not yet. I felt like I was vomiting words into the phone.

Frank said nothing until I was finished. There was a long silence on the phone, and then he said: "Jen, if you don't go and your Mom dies, you'll never forgive yourself. If you go, and she doesn't die, you'll have no regrets."

That was all I needed to hear. It was so simple. My mind became calm. In that instant, I knew he was right. "Thank you Frank, thank you," I said and asked, "Now, what did you need?" He laughed and said it was nothing that he couldn't take care of, and I should figure out what I had to do to get on a plane as soon as possible.

I called my boss and told him what was going on. In typical form, he told me to take as much time as I needed. I had twenty-eight sick days that they cleared me to use in Florida with my mom. Either I would stay the month and come home with my mom renewed, or I would stay with Mom for whatever time she had left, help with the funeral arrangements, and come home after burying her.

I had absolutely no idea how the future was going to unfold. There were too many variables at that moment. As scared as I was of the future, nothing could have prepared me for the unexpected spiritual awakening that transpired over the next twenty days.

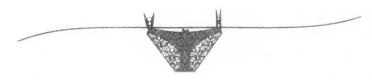

Chapter 25
How You Doin'

I stepped off the plane into the muggy Florida sunshine pouring through the windows at the little Sarasota Airport. My phone rang. It was Max. "Jennifer, I'm in the cell phone lot. I know you checked a bag because your Mom told me you would. So just call me when you get your bag, and I'll pick you up."

I smiled to myself; my mother knew me so well. "Will do Max. See you soon." I hung up the phone and realized I was nervous. In the thirty years that Mom and Max had been together, I honestly did not think that he and I had ever been alone together. What would we talk about?

I left for college soon after they met, and they moved in together my junior year. I'll never forget the phone call I received from Mom letting me know a) they were moving in together, b) she was selling the house, so c) I had to figure out what I wanted to keep and what I wanted to give away of my childhood toys and possessions. It was the first time my mother had occurred to me as a woman who had needs and was going to be moving in with her boyfriend!

Max and I had a good relationship. It wasn't great but it was good. There always seemed to be some tension between us. I attributed it to the fact that he was very quiet and kept to himself, and me, well, I had what people would say is a big personality. People knew when I entered a room even when I didn't say a word.

I had made a pact with myself coming in on the plane that I would tone things down, that I would be quiet, and that I would listen more than I would talk. I promised myself I'd be far more aware of my surroundings than I ever had been before. I wanted to do that for Mom. I also wanted to do that for Max. I could only imagine what he must be feeling.

I picked up my suitcase and went to the car. I had packed the largest suitcase I owned because I wasn't sure how long I was staying. I had no idea what shape my mom was in and whether I'd be staying through the months of March and April, or whether it would be a short trip.

Max pulled up and I loaded my bag into the back of his car. He looked at it, and then at me. "Well I guess you came prepared for everything," he said. I had—for everything but a funeral. I had packed nothing formal or black because I didn't want to be prepared for that at all.

"How's Mom?" I asked.

"You'll see when you get home. She's doing all right," he responded.

"How are you?" I asked, as I put my hand over his.

He looked at me, held my hand for a moment, gave me a sort of smile and said, "I'm all right, I guess."

It was a question I would ask a lot over the next twenty days. It was a question he would begin to ask me a lot. Our entire relationship changed that February. It would change in a way that I never could have predicted and would never have thought would happen had my mom not been ill.

Chapter 26
Paradise in Flamingo Ridge

*I*magine yourself in the Florida heat and sun. Now imagine yourself making a right turn into Flamingo Ridge and immediately the temperature drops by ten or twenty degrees. The people who owned the land stipulated in their will that no vegetation would be cut down. So, Flamingo Ridge boasts seventy-five different types of shrubs and trees. It has a multitude of fresh oranges, grapefruit and avocado. A couple of wild peacocks roam the property, as well. It is like driving into a mythical land when you take that right turn.

The people who live in Flamingo Ridge are quite extraordinary, too. There are so many retired professors that they offer "Flamingo Ridge University" with all types of classes, talks and seminars for people.

There is a library chock-full of books and movies to check out. There are all kinds of art classes—photography, pottery, tap, line dancing, and watercolors, to name a few. There is truly something for everyone. There are multiple swimming pools and water aerobics classes, drinks at sunset, jazz concerts, movies and tennis courts. It was the perfect place for Mom and Max. Max was an avid tennis player and Mom, well, my mom loved everyone and everything so she not only wound up co-leading a tap dance troupe, but started a book club and the 5:00 P.M. Group around their shared pool with snacks and drinks every night at five.

Max dropped me off at their friend Teri's house instead of going right over to their house. He told me there was no rush because Mom knew I was going there first to settle in. Teri was not only a friend but a fellow tap dancer and meticulous with details. Mom relied on her to bring the tape deck and make sure everything ran smoothly for classes.

I walked into Teri's place and my mouth fell open. I felt like I was in a European flat. As it turned out, Teri was an avid international traveler and had led trips all over the world. The furnishings were spectacular, but that was the least of it. Teri lived right on the bay. The entire back wall of her home was made up of sliding glass doors overlooking the bay and the mangrove trees at its shoreline.

I breathed in deeply and felt a connection with the water. My anxiety about seeing Mom immediately dissipated. I'd had a deep love of the water since I was a child. I spent hours on the beach swimming, digging holes, and simply looking out at the ocean and breathing in and out with the tide.

Teri showed me to my room (my very own room and bathroom!) and then gave me a tour of her condo. It was simply lovely. I noticed she had a special nook opposite the bay view where she sat and read *The New York Times*. She also had binoculars and bird books ready to identify species.

"Oh, you get *The New York Times*, that's great," I said.

"I read it every morning with my coffee. We can share tomorrow morning."

As I unpacked my suitcase, Teri came into the bedroom.

"You know, Ellie and I fought over who would have you this week," Teri said. Ellie was a wonderful artist friend of my mother's, and she made gorgeous pottery. "Why are you going somewhere else? Why don't you just stay here while you are in Sarasota? This can be your home," she said.

"You know, my mom never wants to be a burden," I responded. "That's ridiculous," Teri said. "You'll stay here. Why should you move? Why should you have that added stress at this time? Besides, I like the idea of having a roommate; it will give me company, too."

So that was that.

I finished unpacking my bag and asked Teri for a key since I was going to walk over to Mom's place.

"Oh, I don't lock the door. It's always open. I only lock it at night," she said.

"Aren't you afraid someone will break in?" I asked.

"No one ever has and they can have what they want, honestly. I only lock it at night" she replied.

I liked that Teri didn't lock her door. That was one of many things I would grow to love about her. Since my mom didn't get up until around nine a.m., Teri and I would start our day with the strongest coffee I'd ever tasted, buttered Pita bread, and *The New York Times* and *Sarasota Herald*. We read things out loud to one another, passed sections back and forth and commented on recent political events. After I'd return at the end of the day, we'd sit with a glass of wine, talking and watching old black and white classic movies on TV.

Teri and I would sit on her couch and talk for hours. She was fascinating. She was retired but doing so much with her life—tutoring, book club, tap class, water aerobics, and yoga. I loved hearing about her travels around the world and only hoped I could have such a wonderful life by the time I got be in my seventies. Her home became my home during my stay and was a welcome retreat at the end of some very tiring, stressful and uncertain days.

Chapter 27
Not Much Time

I walked through Flamingo Ridge over to Mom and Max's condo. I wasn't sure what to expect. I didn't know how Mom would look. She sounded fine on the phone, but that was my mom. She always sounded fine. I was nervous. I was scared. The one thing I didn't want to say out loud was that I was desperately afraid that this month might be the last time I would see my mom alive.

"Hello," I called out as I entered.

"Hi, Sweetie! I'm in here," my mom called from her office.

I nervously walked into her office, rounded the corner, and saw her grinning from ear to ear. I had to hold back my shock. Although it was my mom and her smile, to me she looked like a talking skeleton. At that moment I knew this would be the end. She had a muddy brown hue to her skin, sort of like brackish swamp water. I can't explain it any other way.

I put all of those thoughts aside as she held out her arms to me and I gave her a big hug and a kiss.

"Awww," she said into my ear. "It's so good to see you."

"Let me get out of here so you two can talk," Max said as he folded up his paper and left the room.

I sat on the small love seat. My mom was in a small recliner so she could stretch herself out in order to get her food down easier. She had a small glass next to her filled with what looked like a milkshake.

"What's that?" I asked.

"That's Ensure," she explained, "I need to count all of my calories so that I can show Dr. F. that I'm getting all the nutrition I need." She had a special notebook next to her and proudly showed me the tiny rows of numbers adding up her calorie count for each day.

She went on to tell me what Dr. F. had told her at the hospital. He would see her again for surgery if that was what she chose to do. He said he'd seen it before. Ovarian cancer spreads to the intestines and creates a blockage. It was only a matter of time before that happened to Mom because the chemotherapy treatments had run their course. At this point my mom had had cancer for nearly four-and-a-half years.

"And if you choose not to have the surgery?" I asked.

"Well that's one option. If I don't have surgery it is only a matter of time until my body shuts down. I'm not ready for that. I'm not ready to go yet. The other option is to find an experimental drug trial. I'm meeting with Dr. S. on Thursday to discuss everything. You'll go with me."

"Experimental drugs?" I asked. My Aunt Jackie had mentioned something in our last conversation. Truthfully, though, in my haste to leave Denver, I hadn't listened very closely.

"I don't want to talk about this anymore. Fill me in on what you've been doing."

We sat and talked, then had some dinner. I watched as Max poured Mom a Coke.

"You're drinking that?" I said with astonishment.

"It helps me burp so I can get the food down," she explained.

I don't remember what we spoke about, but we kept the conversation light. I had a lot more questions I wanted to ask, but I remembered my vow to follow their lead and didn't press the issue.

I went back to Teri's and called Aunt Jackie, as I had promised I would.

"How does she look?" Jackie asked.

"She looks exhausted, weak, and tired," I said.

As it turned out, Mom and Jackie had spoken earlier in the day and discussed options. Jackie told me something my mom had not: it was up to us to find the experimental drug trial. Dr. S. and her staff didn't have time to look through all of the options. Worse than that, with the number of chemo treatments Mom had had—six in all—Dr. S. was not optimistic about being able to find a trial that would accept her. We had three days to find a miracle.

"Jen, there isn't much time," Aunt Jackie said. I gulped and held back my tears. "Okay, we will find an experimental trial. I don't know how we are going to do that. I don't even know where to start, but we will do it," I said to her.

"Well, let's talk tomorrow when you get over to your Mom's. I'll do what I can from here," she said.

I hung up the phone and was very still and silent. As odd as it sounded, I was in my element. There were a lot of times over the last twenty years when I had often been told something was impossible. My usual response was "Oh yeah? Watch this!" I hadn't always been successful, but many times I was. It was the thrill of the game and playing full out no matter the outcome that mattered. In this moment, it was another chance at life, or not. It was Sunday evening, February 6, 2011.

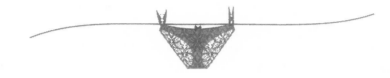

Chapter 29
Dead Woman Tapping

I spent the next twenty-four hours taking a crash course in medical terminology related to cancer, clinical trials and everything associated with them. I now knew the National Institute of Health like the back of my hand. Aunt Jackie kept sending me possible clinical trials from her computer in Massachusetts. My friend Sue connected me with her childhood friend who was the head of the Oncology Department at a major hospital in New York.

I made myself comfortable at the computer in my mom's office, with my Bluetooth on one side of my head and the house phone on the other. I asked Mom questions while she relaxed in her chair, Max sat on the loveseat, and we went through her entire medical history. Max would answer the house phone, bring me things to eat, and encourage me to take a break. The food I could handle, but I wasn't budging until I found a possible clinical trial for Mom. Mom and Max spent their time finding the paperwork I needed, answering questions, or faxing information to various hospitals around the country.

By this point I had a three-ring binder divided into 14 sections. Each section contained a possible clinical trial listing the doctor in charge, possible locations, contact people, and all of the notes I had taken on Monday. That evening I called Aunt Jackie and Uncle Joe and filled them in. Jackie took on communicating to other family members because my phone was ringing off the hook. I had a headache that wouldn't go away, and I couldn't deal with repeating the same story over and over again. We hadn't found the miracle on Monday, but Tuesday would be another day.

I showed up the next morning a bit earlier than usual, wanting to get a start on calling doctor's offices and hospitals. Mom was in her bedroom. It took her a long time to get going in the morning. She came out of her bedroom and into the office a little before eleven.

"You ready to go?" she asked.

"Go where? I've got work to do," I replied.

"To tap class, of course," she answered.

On one hand, I couldn't believe she was going. She was so weak from the little bit of food she was ingesting that she had to hold herself up as she walked from room to room. Watching her eat was painful, to say the least. But I knew how much she loved her tap class, and I wanted to go because she had asked.

Tap class was only a few hundred feet away, but Mom was too tired to walk and it would've taken too long, so I drove her over. The class, being taught by Dixie, was already underway. Ever the teacher, Mom settled in at the front of the room, watching and giving critiques.

"I brought my tap shoes," she told me pulling them from her bag and showing them off proudly.

"You feel good enough to dance with us?" Dixie asked.

"We'll give it a try," she replied.

My heart caught in my throat as I watched my beautiful Mom put on her tap shoes. This was going to be the last time, I thought to myself and kicked myself for not going with her every time she had asked me before. I pushed such thoughts out of my head as soon as they entered; they were useless. My mother got up to tap. As she danced, all I could think was, "Dead Woman Tapping." I nearly laughed out loud. My sense of humor was so inappropriate at times.

I picked up my camera and began taking pictures of her dancing with the troupe. She was dressed in jeans, a brown zip-up sweater, a large scarf wrapped around her neck, and a scarf hiding her disappearing hair. She looked so tiny inside all of those clothes, yet she was the epitome of grace and style.

Her face against the dark brown of her sweater and the suntanned skin of the other Floridians was a chalky white. Her eyes were sunken and she had deep hollows underneath them. The lipstick she had so painstakingly put on her lips and her dark scarf covering what was left of her hair made her skin appear much paler. She simply looked exhausted. Yet, she came to tap class as always and brought me along.

My mother was the consummate performer. She loved being in front of an audience, and had been in community theater performances for as long as I could remember. She came alive when she was in front of people—smiling and exuding a brightness and lightness that no one else on stage seemed to possess.

But today, Mom was not light or bright. She was exhausted. But the show must go on. She never missed a step to the dance she and Dixie had choreographed to *Ain't Misbehavin'*. She didn't miss a beat when it was time to dance to *Singin' in the Rain*, either. And, of course, they had to start in proper form for their upcoming show. It was a show that my mother would never perform in, but we didn't know it at the time.

As I videotaped her dancing to *Ain't Misbehavin'*, I had to stifle my sobs. Tears were running down my face, and I was helpless to stop them. I didn't want her to see me crying. I didn't want her to know that in that moment I had given up hope. I couldn't let her see me that way because I knew it would crush her. I was the one who had told her: "We will find an experimental drug."

Deep down inside, unless something altered dramatically, I knew that this was the last time I would see her dance. No one knew what was coming, but I knew what was predictable.

Chapter 30
There's No Place Like Home

*D*ance class ended, and I drove Mom back to the condo. I got on the phone, and by the end of the day I had organized the pages in a three ring binder. A red tab indicated that Mom had had too many rounds of chemo to qualify. Yellow meant we still had questions to answer. The two or three green tabs were possibilities with options we still had to discuss with Dr. S.

One radical treatment included flying Mom to a hospital in Minnesota where she would have a stem cell transplant harvested from a likely matching donor. I would gladly be her donor. Better yet, my stepbrother Steve and his family lived in Minneapolis and I knew they would be happy to host her while she was in Minneapolis for months at a time during treatment. However, we couldn't figure out how to manage the follow-up visits after she was discharged. The point is we were considering everything.

Then I hit the jackpot. There was a clinical trial a few hours away. The nurse and I had spoken a number of times. The treatment included traditional chemo—the one that Mom had responded to in 2007 during her only remission—as well as an experimental drug. There was a 66% chance she'd get the real drug, and a 33% chance she'd get the placebo, but if she qualified, those odds were better than not doing the experimental drug test at all. The one question that was unanswered was whether the blockage in her intestine was so bad that the oral medication wouldn't be able to do its job. The only way to find out was for Mom to have an MRI. I put in a call, and the nurse said she would call on Wednesday.

On Wednesday, I made more phone calls and wrote more emails because I wasn't going to put all of my eggs in one basket. I wanted Mom to have options. When I finally heard back from the nurse, she told me that the same trial was being held at the local hospital, and the doctor in charge was her own oncological surgeon. I gasped. I was more than pissed off.

"Why didn't he tell my mom that was an option?" I calmly asked the nurse.

"He likely thought she wouldn't qualify because she's had so much chemo," she replied.

"Are you kidding me?" I wanted to scream through the phone. I bit my tongue, but it wasn't easy. I was appalled that he hadn't even asked whether Mom would qualify and simply assumed she wouldn't. I understood where he was coming from, but it was such a different approach to life than I had. I had to remember that I was the one with the weirdly positive attitude. I looked at everything like it was possible, and I kept asking until there was an answer, "Yes."

The nurse told me that we'd have to talk to the doctor and his office would get back to me by Thursday. I told the nurse about our other appointment with Mom's oncologist and asked if she could get back to me sooner, if possible. She said she could.

We walked into the oncologist's office. Mom and Max sat in in the two office chairs while the staff brought in a third chair for me. I was usually very quiet in these meetings and allowed Mom and Max to ask the questions. Mom took meticulous notes in her tiny spiral notebooks. This time was a bit different. Armed with my three-ring binder, I laid out the options and told her about the trial at Sarasota Memorial. She was thrilled and amazed that we had accomplished so much in such a short period of time.

As it turned out, both doctors had already conferred on the matter and were giving Mom a green light to move ahead with the trial at Sarasota Memorial. The next hurdle was to undertake some tests to see how badly the cancer was blocking Mom's intestines. If it was too bad, she couldn't participate because she'd simply regurgitate the experimental drug. Tests were scheduled for that Monday, Valentine's Day. What a perfect gift, I thought.

We left the doctor's office walking on air. We were all so happy, and it was time to celebrate. We went to Mom's favorite vegan restaurant. We all had a cocktail and ordered dinner. A giant weight had been lifted from our shoulders. There were still "what-ifs." Mom had to go in for testing on Monday morning and we wouldn't know the results of those tests immediately. But none of us wanted to talk about that. We were too happy. Nothing could spoil our mood. I saw my mom's face relax for the first time since I arrived and she ate an entire meal. It was a wonderful feeling we had right then, a feeling we hadn't experienced for a while.

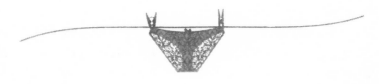

Chapter 31
I Feel Helpless

On Monday, February 14th, we had a very early appointment with the nurse who would be our guide through the testing that could qualify Mom for the experimental drug. We had to walk to various departments throughout the morning. Mom had to sit down often because she was so tired and out of breath. Every time we suggested a wheelchair or offered our hand, she would wave us off. She didn't want our help. It had nothing to do with pride. It was simply her way of telling herself, and us, that she was okay.

The nurse settled us into the radiology unit. Mom's job was to drink a few bottles of barium to get ready for the MRI. The nurse brought her the first bottle with a straw. Mom's shaking hand reached out for it.

She was very worried about drinking the barium because she had had problems before. The stuff looked like a thick milkshake and tasted like chalk but was necessary so the MRI could show the appropriate images of her internal organs.

"I'm really nervous about drinking this. I could barely keep it down the last time I had to have it," she said. "It tastes just awful, and I wasn't having problems with my digestion then." She smiled at me, but it was a tense sort of smile that did little to hide the nervousness she felt. I smiled back at her.

"It will be okay Mom, you'll see." You can do this, I thought to myself, but I was holding my breath. I'd never seen Mom this scared. Max and I took turns sitting next to Mom, coaxing her to drink the thick, chalky liquid. She was having a tough time; she was burping periodically and holding her stomach.

"What if I can't drink it all? I won't be able to have the MRI and we won't get into the experimental trial," she said to me. "You worked so hard to find this." She was pale. She was gaunt. She looked like a little girl—her eyes wide, wanting us to tell her everything was going to be okay and I did, but didn't believe my own words. I turned my head away to hide the tears that started rolling down my cheeks.

"It'll be okay, Red," said Max, using one of his pet names for her. He took her hand and patted it. She snatched it away from him and waved him off. She hadn't been able to be touched for a long time.

She took another sip and put the bottle down. She was silent.

Then she looked at me, fear pouring out of her eyes.

"I have to throw up," Mom said in the smallest voice I'd ever heard. I sprung up, and got a garbage pail for her. I helplessly watched her throw up.

"It's only a little bit," she said after a few moments. "I think I'm okay."

"Want me to ask the nurse if they have Strawberry flavored Barium? At least that's your favorite flavor."

"Yeah, honey, why don't you do that," she said with a sad smile.

I did ask the nurse, but the only flavor was chocolate. I reported back to my mom who already had the straw back in her mouth.

"It's okay, I'll deal with it."

I decided to call the nurse who had helped us earlier in the day because she had been able to calm her down. I told her what was happening. She wasn't available but could send her assistant.

"Anything that you can do for my mom. Anything at all would be wonderful," I said.

I sat down across from Mom and Max. I wasn't sure what the heck to do. I felt so incredibly alone and helpless. What could I do for her? My thoughts were interrupted.

"I have to throw up again." Max reached down to hand Mom the wastebasket. Mom threw up. Then she threw up again. And again, and again. She couldn't stop. I silently watched her convulse and spew out the thick liquid in the anonymous black wastebasket.

I sat there feeling afraid and useless. Tears sprang into my eyes. I took deep breaths trying to will them away – Mom didn't need to see me upset. But once they started I couldn't stop them. I took another look at Mom, and Max sitting next to her holding her hand and mumbled, "I'll be right back." I sprang from my chair and walked out of the hospital. As soon as I heard the doors close behind me I started sobbing uncontrollably in the bright sunshine as I walked blindly down the street with no idea where I was going. I passed other patients and nurses and doctors. Oh, God, what do I do? What do I do? Somebody help me. Somebody give me an answer. What do I do? I just kept chanting this mantra over and over again in my mind.

I stopped at the corner and my friend Betty's voice came to mind. "If you need anything, anything at all, you call me." She had just lost her

husband after a prolonged illness and knew what I was going through.
Please oh please oh please oh please be home. Please pick up the phone.
I said to myself as I rang her phone number.

"Hello?" she said as she picked up the phone.

"Betty, its Jen. Can you talk?" I asked.

"Of course, what's going on?" she asked.

I told her where I was, what we were doing. I told her that I couldn't
let my mom see me so upset because it would upset her even more. I
told her that I had just walked out. I told her how scared and alone I
felt, and how I had what seemed like a never-ending headache ever since
I arrived. I told her about how brave my mom was, and how tired she
was. Betty just listened and listened and listened, until I thought I had
nothing more to say.

"Anything else?" she asked.

"I want my mom to live. I want her to be able to get these tests. I
want her qualified for the trial. I want a miracle. I want to stop crying."

"You may never stop crying, Jennifer. It's part of the grieving
process. You are grieving your Mom now, even while she is living. You
are grieving how your relationship used to be. It's all okay. It's okay to be
scared. It's okay to want her to live. It's okay to want a miracle because
you truly don't know how this all is going to end."

I really heard what she said and I got it was okay to be all over the
place. I also recognized that while we don't know how things are going
to end, truth is we do. We all die in the end. We just don't know when.
Maybe we should be more scared all the time so that we stop taking
life for granted and remember to celebrate every moment we have. I
breathed in deeply.

"Betty, thank you. I am going to celebrate every moment. Mom will
either qualify for the tests or not. She'll either get the experimental drug,
or not. It will work, or it won't. And I can celebrate every moment of her
life up to the end. I can do that." Relief washed over me because I had

stopped thinking about what might happen and simply started living right there, right then, and right in that moment.

"Beautiful Jen. Just beautiful. Thank you for reaching out and for being there for your Mom." I hung up the phone. I was calm. I was peaceful. The outcome didn't matter. The only thing that mattered was expressing my unconditional love for my mom in this moment. That was it.

I walked back into the hospital. The nurses were taking Mom back to the MRI.

"Hi honey. They say they can do the tests without me drinking the Barium, isn't that great," she said and smiled at me. She looked so relieved.

"Yeah, Mom, that's great," I said as I kissed her on the cheek.

I watched the nurses wheel her away. Max stood up to go, but they told him he should stay behind. He gave her a kiss on the cheek and returned to the waiting room chair across from me.

"Where did you go?" he asked.

"I started crying and couldn't stop and didn't want Mom to see me that way and so I went outside. I couldn't take it," I whispered. He looked at me with tears in his eyes and took my hand. "I know exactly what you mean. I get that way, too."

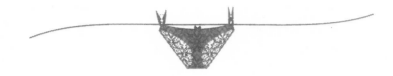

Chapter 32
Emergency Room Visit

*L*ater that afternoon, I dropped Mom and Max off at their condo. We were all relieved to have gotten through the harrowing experience of the barium and MRI successfully. We were hopeful that the pictures would enable the nurses and doctors to see what they needed to see, but we didn't know for sure if they would. Still, we were on pins and needles waiting to hear from the nurse in a few days.

I drove back over to Teri's house. While I was able to take a month off from work, there were still matters I needed to tend to and emails I needed to answer. I also had to call Aunt Jackie and Uncle Joe with an update. As I spoke to them, Teri appeared in my doorway frantically waving her arms.

"Max is on the house phone. He needs you at the condo right away. Your Mom started throwing up again."

I quickly hung up and raced over to the condo. I felt like I was in the middle of the movie Groundhog Day, where the day's events just repeat and repeat. I was panicky, sweaty, nervous, sick to my stomach, and already crying.

"Hello?" I said as I walked in the door.

"We're in here," Max called out to me.

"I'm okay, I'm okay. I don't know why you came," said my mom as she got back into bed.

"What's going on?"

"Your Mom started throwing up again so I called Dr. F.'s office."

"What did he say," I asked. I didn't know if this was simply a result of leftover nerves from the day or whether we had more to worry about.

Mom had hated being babied over the last five years. While she wasn't well at that moment, she certainly wasn't going to let anyone talk for her.

"I'm fine. The doctor said as long as I can keep some food down today and I don't throw up again, I can go into his office tomorrow. He just wants to make sure I didn't hurt myself today with all of the throwing up," she said as she slid under the covers of her bed.

"Well I guess it's a false alarm. I think your Mom should go to the emergency room, but she doesn't want to," said Max. We talked a bit more, but in the end Mom's opinion won out as it always did. Our goal was always to listen to her and respect her wishes. She rarely showed she was in pain or complained, and she was always smiling. I honestly didn't know how she did it.

I left and went back to Teri's. I don't remember what I did for the rest of the day, but I do remember the call I received around eight or nine that night.

"Come on, we are going to the Emergency Room," Max said on the phone. "Your Mom hasn't stopped throwing up since she ate supper."

"Did you call an ambulance?" I asked.

"Your Mom doesn't want one. She doesn't want people to think the worst so you come with her car, and we'll get her there."

I drove to their condo and ran around the car to open the passenger door. Max helped Mom get gingerly into the car. She dragged a garbage can lined with a plastic bag into the back seat with her in case she threw up again. Dr. F.'s prediction that he would see my mom again came true, though the timing wasn't what he had in mind. Instead of a few weeks or a month, it was exactly one week since she had left the hospital the last time.

By this time, we had been in the emergency room for a few hours. Mom was once again in a wheelchair groaning and doubled over in pain. She had thrown up her pain medication much earlier and they wouldn't give her an IV for the pain until she was admitted. She didn't want to be touched so I couldn't even rub her back to soothe her the way she used to for me when I was a child.

She simply sat in the chair with her head in her hand. Her face was gaunt and gray, matching the color of her gray velour sweatshirt. If she hadn't been so sick, she would've liked the fact that she was color coordinated.

"Oooohhhh. I'm sorry honey for moaning. It just hurts so much," Mom said.

That was my mom – apologizing for making others feel uncomfortable even if she couldn't help it. She didn't want anything about the cancer to make us uncomfortable, so we never truly knew the amount of pain that she was in.

Around midnight, they finally wheeled her into an examining room and hooked her up to intravenous fluids for pain medication and nourishment. After about ten minutes Mom got this goofy grin on her face.

"Happy Mommy!" she said gleefully.

"Oh, I'm so glad, Mom," I said with tears in my eyes.

Max was silent sitting next to me. He was the one who, for the last four-and-a-half years, had taken care of my mother. He'd been to every doctor's appointment and every chemo session.

"Storti," he began.

"Yes, Toffler my love," my mom said as she beamed back at him.

The two of them were so cute together and their love so strong. They'd been calling each other by their last names for as long as I could remember. I don't know how or why it started, but I had joined in the fun years ago. Every time I called and he answered the phone I'd say, "Toffler? It's Coken."

"We need to talk about this surgery, Storti," he said.

I was surprised he was so candid. It was something my mom did not want to talk about. She didn't want surgery because she was afraid of what they might find. She didn't want to be told how much time she had left. I was proud of him for bringing it up.

"I don't want to talk about it," Mom stated.

"Well it seems like we have no choice. Dr. F. said you'd likely have to have the surgery, and now's the time," Max came back.

Mom got tears in her eyes, and her lip started trembling.

"What if they tell me that there is nothing that they can do?" she asked softly.

"Then that's what they'll tell you," said Max.

Max wasn't trying to be callous. He was just a matter of fact kind of guy. He'd been a window shade salesman for thirty years in Cleveland spending his days measuring people's windows. He was a facts and figures kind of guy.

Emboldened by Max's forthrightness, I said "Mom we don't know what will happen if they do the surgery. We won't know how bad things are until after the doctor opens you up. Either he can take out the diseased part and give you more time, or we invite the rest of the kids, grandkids, and great grandkids to say goodbye."

"Jen's right, you know. I think you need to do the surgery so we know what we are dealing with don't you Storti?" said Max.

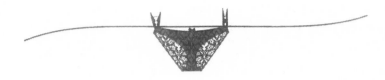

Chapter 33
No More Living in Limbo

*m*om looked at us both blankly. Max got up to go find the bathroom. It was just my mom and me in the emergency room. She was staring at me and was very, very quiet. She got tears in her eyes. "I'm not ready to go yet," she said. "I'm scared."

I swallowed hard. I'd been waiting for the right moment to talk to her about the inevitable, and this seemed like the right time. I knew I had been walking on eggshells worried about the future. I hadn't been living every day freely, appreciating what we had, and focusing on celebrating every day of the life my mom still had left. I knew she hadn't either.

"Mom, you know how you've been asking the angels to keep the traffic light green near home so you don't have to wait?" I asked. ("Oh geez," I thought, "I sound ridiculous.") But I kept going.

"Well, the angels are here to help with big stuff, too. You can ask them to take away your fear and to comfort you. You can talk to them and ask them to protect you through the surgery. They are here to help you in any way. You just need to ask."

My mom nodded in agreement. "I guess I forgot about that," she said.

It was amazing to me that Mom and I could now have this kind of conversation. Before she had been diagnosed with cancer, she didn't believe in anything other than what she could see, taste, touch, or smell.

"It's not that I don't believe in a higher power. I just would like proof," she used to tell me.

"Mom, even if you leave us on this physical plane, you will still be with us. Every time I see the color yellow, I will think of you. I will hear your words when I am faced with making hard decisions. I will find joy in dance and performance that you instilled in me since I was young. You are part of me in the way I think about others. You've made such a profound impact on my life that you will never go away." Both of our eyes filled with tears.

"Your friends feel the same way. You should hear the wonderful things they've been telling me about you. You have no idea how much you are a part of each of us. So, while your physical body may leave us, you will live on in each of our lives so you really will never have left us."

As I was saying all of this, my entire left side was warm and vibrating. I had come to trust that when that happened, God, Spirit, Christ Consciousness – whatever your own version is – was speaking through me. My mom sighed.

"Honey, I know you're right, but I'll miss this—this right here, us sharing and seeing each other and hugging each other. I'll miss the physical plane," Mom said.

I looked into the hollow sockets of my mother's eyes. I lingered over her beautiful porcelain skin, not a wrinkle at age 70. Today she was gray with fear and exhaustion.

"I get it Mom. I know you are scared. I am too. The honest truth is you are going to die." She gasped. I swallowed hard. "We are *all* going to die Mom. It's the one terminal illness none of us can escape. From the moment we are born, we start dying. No one remembers this because if we sat around and only thought about the fact that we were going to die, nothing would be achieved. What would be the point? So we forget, and we go about our lives and become amazing scientists and bankers, Moms and Dads, chefs, carpenters, school teachers and geologists. In the forgetting, we take a stand for civil rights and ending hunger, and we find new ways to teach kids with learning disabilities. We discover the theory of relativity and penicillin. This is life – the forgetting so we can give it our all, and the remembering to be grateful for what we have, give thanks and ask for more."

My heart was in my throat, my hands were shaking, and my voice was trembling. I had never spoken to my mom about her death before. I had always avoided it because I thought by speaking about it I'd make it more real or bring death more quickly to her. But I knew that what I was saying was exactly what needed to be said in that moment.

I continued, "There are only two dates on a tombstone, Mom: the date you are born, and the date you die, and there is a dash in the middle. Life is about that dash. Life is about living in the dash, living the best way you know possible so that when it comes time to put the end date on, you can say you gave it your all. But you have stopped living in the dash, Mom. You have been living to avoid that end date on your tombstone. Do you want to live the rest of your days, or months, or years in trepidation hoping that the end date doesn't come too soon? Or do you want to live your life as you always have—loving everyone unconditionally, seeing the beauty in everything, and adoring your family. How do you want to live the rest of your life, Mom? Because it's time. It's time for you to choose. I want you to live in that dash, Mom. I want you to celebrate every moment you have left. If you have the surgery, and we have fifteen days to celebrate how incredible you are, then we have fifteen days. If it's more, it's more, but at least we'll know. But you have to choose to live in the dash Mom, I can't make that choice for you."

My mom was just stared at me wide-eyed while I spoke. I had one more thing to say.

"However, Mom you can choose to live or you can choose to go. Because if you are too tired – tired of all of this chemo and throwing up and regulating your diet and the pain – if you are so tired that you are ready to go, you just let me know. I will support that choice, and I will stay and help you with your transition and be with Max. If you want to live, I will support that choice and I will stay as long as you want and get you through the surgery and beyond. But how you've been living? Barely living because you are so afraid to die? It's not living at all. It's like you've been holding your breath for months, waiting for the bad news or the end. It is time to choose: life or death, but no limbo anymore. I won't have it."

Mom continued to be quiet. I had said a lot and knew she needed time to process. At that precise moment Max walked back into the room, so I didn't get a chance to hear Mom's reaction. Through the years, my relationship had grown into the kind where we could say anything to each other. However, I'd never had the courage to talk so plainly to her about her death. I was proud of myself for my honesty and I hoped I hadn't gone overboard.

We said goodbye to Mom around two in the morning as they finally wheeled her to a room in the hospital. Both of her doctors would see her in the morning and surgery was scheduled for a few days later. Mom looked scared and small, but at least she was in a place to get care so Max and I could go and sleep through the night. I kissed her pale, gray face goodnight and smoothed her hair.

"Goodnight, Mamasan. I love you," I said.

"I love you, too, sweetheart," she responded.

"Veeerrrrry much," we both said at the same time.

Max and I walked silently back to the car.

"That must have been really hard to talk about the surgery, Max," I said.

"Yep," was his response.

I put my hand over his and squeezed. He looked at me with a smile and a few tears sprang up in his eyes. He started the car and we drove home.

Chapter 35
483!!!

The next morning, I walked into Mom's hospital room at about eleven o'clock. Max had taken the morning shift and had been there reading the paper. He wasn't in the room at the time, however. I looked at Mom and she smiled a wide smile. Her face was flushed with good health and there was a glow about her. Her eyes were bright and there were no more hollows under her sockets.

There was a halo of pale yellow light surrounding her. It expanded beyond her body and encompassed the hospital bed, her bedside table and extended up and out, touching the ceiling and the walls. There was a sparkle in the air. In that moment I knew.

"You chose, didn't you, Mom? You chose to live!" I exclaimed.

She smiled with recognition. "Yeah, I guess I did."

Mom had the surgery a few days later. Max and I spent hours in the waiting room holding hands, reading the paper, pacing about, and drinking coffee. I had my computer with me so I could give real time updates to my Aunt Jackie. When the doctor came out, he gave us an update. He had had to remove sections of her bowel in two places. He thought he had it all, but he was very upfront with us.

"All I've done is slow down the growth of the cancer. It will return to her bowel at some point. But she has a lot more time now, and we can be assured that when she recovers from the surgery she'll be able to digest the experimental drug." That was the best news I'd heard since my arrival.

We were able to see Mom that afternoon and decided on who was going to come in the morning. Max would take the morning shift so he could bring more of Mom's stuff over. I would take lunch and the afternoon shift, then Max would join me and we'd get dinner then say goodnight to Mom together. We were in for a pretty lengthy recovery time—at least a few weeks at the hospital and then in-home treatment of the wound.

The next morning after working out, I received a phone call from Mom. I could tell she was pretty high on her pain medication. She was slurring her words a bit and acting pretty giddy. I was having trouble understanding her.

"Mom, I'll be there in an hour or so. Why don't we talk when I get there?" I asked. It was pretty cute to hear her so stoned.

"Okay, honey," she paused. "Honey? Leggings," she added.

"Leggings, Mom?" I asked.

"Leggings. I don't know what I wanted to say about leggings but remind me when you get here," she said.

I giggled as I hung up the phone. What a goofball. It was nice to smile for a change as I thought about my mom. I had been holding my breath for the last two weeks. I realized in that moment I was holding it again. I let it out and took a deep breath in.

I had created an awesome support network. My cross-fit trainer and the group I trained with back home had agreed to Skype me into the workout sessions a few mornings a week. I had no camera on my computer, so thankfully they couldn't see my spandex self-magnified in front of a video camera. But I could see them, and it was a wonderful thing to have some semblance of normalcy. I pushed myself as hard as I could, took a shower and headed to the hospital.

"Jeffner!" my mom exclaimed as I came in, using my childhood nickname. She held out her arms for a hug and a kiss.

I went to her to get my hug, careful not to trip on the IV or press too intensely on the surgery site. I filled her in on my morning, and she began to tell me about something that had happened in the middle of the night.

"I wouldn't tell this to anyone else but you, honey. But I think I woke up in the middle of the night and went to the bathroom, although how I could get myself out of bed I don't know. But when I woke up, there were fine art paintings hanging on the wall, all of them masterpieces, and I could step in and out of them. I spent a few hours in each of the paintings. I don't know for how long," she said.

"Well that must've been kind of cool to be able to do that." I said smiling to myself. Humor the person on drugs, I thought.

Out of seemingly nowhere my mom blurted out "483!"

"Uh, okay, Rainman. What about 483?" I asked, chuckling. She was so cute.

"I don't know, just 483 and the surgery," she responded.

Hmmm, I thought to myself. 483. Maybe I should Google the number on the browser of my smartphone, so I did. The top three sites that popped up with the number 483 in the header referenced an early writing tool used by Socrates. However, when I clicked through to the

Wikipedia entries to find out more, the number itself disappeared. Instead I saw information referencing plot twists in books and movies. It gave an example of Luke Skywalker finding out that Darth Vader is his father. When that was revealed, the story took on a new meaning and went in a new direction.

Well this story certainly took a twist. I had flown to Florida fairly certain Mom was about to die, and I would be leaving knowing we had more time. She had chosen to have the surgery, to live and because of that she could take the experimental drug and our lives were headed in a very different direction. We still didn't know how much time Mom had but we had all chosen to live each day celebrating life. It's funny, to this day, no matter how hard I try to find those references when I Google "483" none of them pop up. I know it was just spirit giving us confirmation of what had happened. By the way Mom also finally gave me her leggings. Nothing special. Just a pair of black leggings that she knew she was never going to wear. Such a practical person was she.

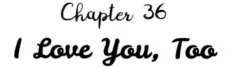

Chapter 36
I Love You, Too

spent most of the month of February with Mom. My days became routine. Since Max took the morning shift, I'd have coffee and toast with Teri and read *The New York Times*. When she wasn't home I'd sit and stare at the blueness of the water. Sometimes I'd cry. Sometimes I'd just focus on breathing in and out. I'd answer a few work emails, workout via Skype with my cross-fit buddies, go for a walk, or run on the beach. I'd show up at the hospital with my lunch just before noon and spend the afternoon with Mom. Around suppertime, Max would arrive and we'd go out for dinner and then return to the hospital together to spend a few more hours with Mom before heading home.

It was during one of those early dinners that my relationship with Max changed forever. It's a funny story how Mom and Max met. I actually introduced them when I was 15 years old. As far back as I can remember we were involved in Community Theater. Either all of us were performing, or my mom and dad were performing, or my mom was performing.

My mom, brother and I were in a local production of "Anything Goes." I was a general cast member, my brother was part of the tech crew and my mom, as usual, was part of the dance troupe. There was a local piano bar and restaurant where the musical director played piano and sang on most nights. Many of the cast members would go, so it became a stop for us to get a bite after a show.

This particular evening was a Jewish holiday. Mom and I had gone to services and stopped by for dinner. Later on we sat around the piano bar and sang songs with the musical director. This was back in the days when smoking was allowed in bars.

I had always been pretty gregarious. I saw a handsome guy across the way that was waving the smoke out of his eyes. He was about my mom's age.

"If the smoke is bothering you, there's no smoke over here," I called out and pointed to a seat next to my mom. Next thing I knew, Max sat down next to her. The rest is history.

Since I left for college at the age of sixteen, I never really "grew up" with Max. Nonetheless, he was a big influence on my life. The thing about Max was he was a pretty quiet and reserved kind of guy, until he had a martini. Then he became tender and silly and would giggle and joke with my mom. Unfortunately, I didn't see that side of him very often because I didn't see him very often; but what we had been going through together that month—the worries, the fears, the laughs, and the tension, day in and day out—had brought us closer together and broken through something, something unspoken until that night.

So there we sat, he with his martini with extra olives, and I with a glass of white wine. We were both very quiet – and contemplative.

"You know Jen, there's something I want to say. I used to dread your visits. You were always so loud, so busy, it seemed like you'd swoop in like this ball of energy and couldn't sit still for a moment. But I know you and your Mom have always been very close, so of course I'd put up with it. I'd just make myself scarce until it was time for dinner."

My heart stopped. I wasn't quite sure where this was going. Max was still looking down at his hands, so I waited.

"This visit has been different. You've been very calm. I don't know what or how you've changed, but you' have done it. And I want to say thank you, and I appreciate you for that. I don't know what I would've done if you hadn't been here. Whatever has gone on in the past is the past. It's done and we have a new relationship, now."

He looked up at me with tears in his eyes and took my hand. I had tears in my eyes too. There was so much I could say at that moment, but few words were needed.

"It has been different, hasn't it? Thank you for saying what you did. The past is the past and we'll start fresh and new. I love you, Max."

"I love you too, Jen."

That was the first time that Max ever told me he loved me. In all those years, he had simply said, "Thank you," when I uttered those three words to him, so I had stopped saying it. What was the point if someone just says thank you? I realized I had given up expressing an honest emotion to him all this time. I wasn't saying I love you to get him to say it back, I was saying I love you because it was true for me. Since that dinner over a year ago, I always end my conversations with Max by telling him I love him. Sometimes he says thank you. But more often than not he says, "I love you, too."

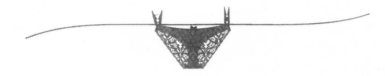

Chapter 37
The Robe

As the month of February drew to a close, I could tell it was time for me to move on. I knew I could have stayed in Sarasota for a few more months – it would have been so easy, and I had already arranged it with my job. But I also intuitively knew that it was time for Mom to move on. It was time for her to rekindle her friendships. She hadn't really called or spoken to anyone but Max and me in nearly a month, with the exception of one or two very close (or very pushy, as Max would say) friends. She had chosen to live; now it was time to start living.

I walked into her hospital room one morning. Our routine was pretty much the same. Mom and I sat and talked while she crocheted.

We always took a walk and did laps around the hospital so Mom could get her strength back. She was so amazing. She had started walking just a day or so after her major surgery.

"Mom, I think it's time for me to go. It's time for you to get back into your life and start relying on your community again."

She looked at me and we both got tears in our eyes. I honestly didn't want to leave her side but somehow knew that she needed to be around her friends. I couldn't stay indefinitely, as much as we both wanted me to. It seemed that the best approach was for her and Max to get back to their "normal" routine and lean on her awesome support system right there in Sarasota. She and Max had so many terrific friends, and they both wanted to see them. But we had cocooned ourselves in the last month. We'd been scared out of our wits and had hunkered down as we figured out the future. Now that things were looking much better, it was time to get into life and time for me to go. We both knew it.

Mom sighed. "I knew this was coming. I knew it. I don't want you to go, but I know it's time."

We talked about who she would call. She really didn't like people seeing her "sick" because she didn't want people treating her any differently or feeling sorry for her. She had such a positive attitude nearly all the time, and she needed everyone around her to be positive. It wasn't the easiest thing to do sometimes.

We spoke about some of the things she would need, like voluminous pants and tops so as not to irritate the surgery site. She also wanted a new bathrobe. Hers was a bit tattered and she loved being put together all the time. She was a beautiful woman who didn't need a lot of makeup. But through all of her time with cancer, including being in the hospital, she made certain to put on her makeup, neatly drawing in the eyebrows she had lost, and donning a wig and hat that matched her outfit.

Mom had a terrific fashion sense. She had even appeared in a local fashion show. I thought it was funny because, once upon a time, getting dressed for work in the morning would give Mom a headache.

Mom had been a schoolteacher for most of my childhood. She and my dad got divorced when I was in junior high, and she realized she wouldn't be able to afford to keep our house on a teacher's salary, even though my dad was helping out. It was important to the two of them that my brother and I be able to stay in the house we'd been living in, so Mom chose to stop teaching and began working for the government in 1976. She worked for the Navy as civilian personnel. Eventually she worked for and ultimately retired from NASA as an education specialist. Her job was to train teachers to use NASA's space curriculum to make math and science more appealing to inner city kids.

I remember sitting on Mom's bed in seventh or eighth grade while she got ready for work. She couldn't figure out what to wear. I loved her clothes. I pulled out a sweater and skirt.

"What about this?" I asked.

"Yeah? That goes together. What shoes should I wear?"

I pulled out my favorite purple suede booties and told her to wear those with tights.

She got dressed and looked simply amazing. That night she and I sat in her closet while I showed her different possibilities of outfits. She actually wrote them down on index cards and kept them in her closet so that she didn't have to think of what to wear in the morning. Nowadays, I was the one getting fashion tips from her!

We talked about the bathrobe she wanted. She was very precise about everything, and her bathrobe was no exception. It had to have the same length and sleeve length as the old one because she was often cold. She wanted something bright and cheerful, and she wanted a nylon robe because not only was she cold, but she had bouts of getting hot from all of the medication she was taking.

I was on a mission. We decided upon loungewear because the fabrics would be softer over the surgery site. We also decided that if the clothes fit me, they would be the right size for Mom. I was a boxers and t-shirt kind of gal, but there I was with the personal shoppers in Neiman Marcus and Nordstrom trying on the latest in soft loungewear, like a real lady. I'd bring the clothes to her hospital room for her to see. I'd model them, and she would give the thumbs up or thumbs down. Then I'd return what she didn't like and look for new things.

It was easier to find the loungewear than the perfect bathrobe. I knew how much time she was going to spend in it, and I wanted it to be beautiful, just like her. It couldn't be just any robe. I went to department store after department store. I tried Sears. I tried Macy's. I even tried maternity stores – what the heck? But I found nothing. All of the robes they carried had short sleeves because the stores were stocking summer clothes.

It was on a last trip back to Macy's to return some items that I saw *the robe*. It was absolutely stunning, just like Mom. It had a white background with flowers in hues of deep purple, burnt orange and other fall colors. It would go perfectly with Mom's red hair. The length was perfect, the sleeves were perfect, and it even gathered in the back.

I took it to the hospital, and Mom's eyes lit up like it was Christmas. She struggled to stand up. She slipped her bony arms into the sleeves, wrapped the silk around her body and gingerly tied the sash over her distended belly. "Take me for a walk," she ordered sashaying her hips at me. "I want to show off this robe!"

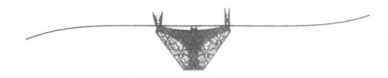

Chapter 38
Not Sticks But Stones

I had made one more necessary stop along the way on my quest for the robe: Elysian Fields. This was the metaphysical bookstore in town and was a favorite stop for Mom and me every time I visited.

When Mom told me she and Max were moving to Florida, my first reaction was: "Great, just what Florida needs, more old Jews driving slowly." Florida was the last place on my list I would want to live. I knew it only from spending a week there every year with my grandparents on spring break, along with every other Jewish kid I knew. It was hot so everyone stayed inside. I loved the outdoors and couldn't bear to be cooped up. My skin was so fair that I couldn't stay outside long before getting sunburned. Not only could I count on an annual visit with my grandparents, I could count on an annual sunburn and my annual bath in tea—supposedly to take the sting out of the sunburn. That's the only Florida I knew.

I had now come to know Sarasota as a very spiritual place. Mom had a good friend, Barbara, who lived downstairs from her back in Cleveland. Barbara and her husband Michael moved to Florida before Mom and Max. In fact, they had enticed my parents to come to Sarasota. Barbara was an angel. She always had a twinkle in her eye and was very connected to spiritual people and places. She had introduced Mom to Elysian Fields, to an alternative therapy center and to the Center for Spiritual Awareness and the powerhouse Reverend Duffy Rutledge. Barbara had been a most welcome guide to my mom as she walked her spiritual journey.

Elysian Fields had all types of book by famous Hay House authors like Wayne Dyer, Mike Dooley and Doreen Virtue. There were such topics as Native American healing, Feng Shui, and the healing power of crystals, for example. The store hosted local tarot card readers and local speakers on spiritual topics. They also carried crystals, gorgeous jewelry, clothing, and other gifts that held uplifting sayings.

Since I knew I was leaving, I wanted to buy some things for Mom to assist her in integrating back into her life. I went to the store not knowing exactly what to get her, but I trusted that Spirit was guiding me there.

I walked into the store and took a deep breath. I walked over to a display case of large crystals, closed my eyes and asked Spirit for guidance. I put my hand up in front of me, palm facing the case. I felt a pressure pushing it down and to the right. I opened my eyes. My hand was hovering over a perfect red jasper wand. It had a cylindrical shape and fit perfectly in to the palm of my hand. It was smooth and was a beautiful mix of light and dark reds, streaks of brown and white quartz running through it, and topped with some green at the tip.

As I picked it up, it felt as if it were pulsating in my hand. I knew it was the perfect piece. I didn't know much about its healing properties, but I trusted my intuition. At the same time, I also was practical and curious, so I used my Smartphone to find out whether my intuition was correct. On Caryl Haxworth's website "Charms of Light" (www. charmsoflight.com) it said: "Red Jasper is gently stimulating and also an extremely protective stone. It can neutralize radiation and other forms of environmental and electromagnetic pollution. Red Jasper rectifies unjust situations and grounds energy. Brings problems to light and provides insights into difficult situations. An excellent 'worry bead,' Red Jasper calms the emotions. Aids in dream recall. Cleans and stabilizes the aura. A stone of health, Red Jasper strengthens and detoxifies the circulatory system, blood and liver."

Okay, that was perfect but I wasn't done yet. There were a few more things to get. I wasn't certain of everything, but I did know that I wanted to get Mom an angel. We were both big readers of Doreen Virtue's book on Angels and used her book *Angel Numbers 101* all the time.

I closed my eyes again and asked Spirit to guide me. When I opened them, they fell on a bin of stones. One in particular drew my attention. It was a small angel made out of smoky quartz. The label read "Archangel Michael." Well that was perfect! Who better to protect my mommy than a statute of Archangel Michael—the most powerful archangel of them all?

Again I consulted Caryl Haxworth's website and this is what it said about smoky quartz: "Smoky Quartz is an excellent grounding stone. It gently neutralizes negative vibrations and is detoxifying on all levels, prompting elimination of the digestive system and protecting against radiation and electromagnetic smog. Smoky Quartz disperses fear, lifts depression and negativity. It brings emotional calmness, relieving stress and anxiety. Promotes positive thoughts and action, and alleviates suicidal tendencies. Dispels nightmares and manifests your dreams.

Smoky Quartz aids concentration and assists in communication difficulties."

Again, perfect. What else? For the third time I closed my eyes and asked for Spirit's guidance. I had already spent time at Elysian Fields on two earlier visits and didn't really "need" anything else. Yet, I sensed that whatever else there was for me to find, it would be for me, not Mom. I was drawn to the book section. I wandered over and began to drift to a variety of texts, until I came to the section of books by Doreen Virtue. The top shelf had multiple copies of her books lined up, except in one place. There, one copy of her book *The Lightworker's Way: Awakening Your Spiritual Power to Know and Heal* was staring at me. That was it!

I took all of my purchases up to the register. The woman behind the counter picked up Doreen Virtue's book, took a good long look at it and began turning it over in her hand.

"Where did you get this?" she asked.

"Right on the shelf with her other books" I responded.

"I've been working here twelve years and know every inch of the store. I've never, ever seen this book before. Are there others?"

"No, it was your only copy."

She smiled at me. "Guess you were supposed to have it."

I smiled to myself. Yep, I guess I was.

I drove back to the hospital to show Mom the jasper wand and the statue of Archangel Michael. I told her how to use them—to sleep with the angel next to her bed, and to hold the wand in her hand over the surgery site while envisioning healthy cells coursing through her veins.

A month or so after Mom was discharged from the hospital, she was on the phone with a dear friend of mine, a gifted psychic from Colorado. Mom was a bit of a skeptic but was willing to try anything.

After her first session, Mom called. She was excited because while on the phone together, my friend had told her to make sure to use the jasper wand that I had bought for her.

"Do exactly what Jennifer told you to do. Hold it in your hand and imagine clean cells coursing through your veins. Imagine the surgery site healing quickly."

My mom said her jaw dropped at that point and she asked her whether I had told her that about the stones I bought and, if not, how did she know about them.

"Jan, I'm psychic, remember?" she giggled in response.

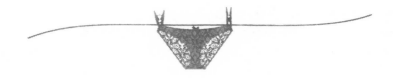

Chapter 38
We Didn't Get A Fair Trial

Mom left the hospital the first week of March 2011. She was able to get regular nursing care at home, which she needed to change her bandages. I took a look at her wound, and it was pretty impressive. She had an incision from "stem to stern"—from her breastbone to the top of her pubic bone. The surgeon had removed about six feet of her intestine then used heavy-duty staples to close up the incision. It was hard for Mom to get comfortable at almost anytime of the day or night. Because her intestines had to remain relatively quiet for healing, she was on a restricted diet. She had to be able to have the strength and stamina for her body to undergo more chemo and the experimental drug.

She was finally able to start the trial the first week of April. It consisted of seven weeks of chemo, one session per week. It was administered in a five-hour drip along with an oral experimental medication. There were a couple of problems with the experimental trial. First of all we had no idea if Mom would be getting the experimental drug or the placebo. There was only a 66% chance she'd get the experimental drug but we liked those odds compared to doing nothing. Second, since she was getting seven weeks of the trial, we'd have no knowledge whether it was working until the latter part of May. At that point she would get another MRI. If the MRI showed no signs of the cancer growth, she could remain on the trial. If at any time there was any indication of cancer growth, Mom would be asked to leave the trial.

So, our fingers were crossed, and we hoped for the best. It was during this time that Mom's friend Judy died. She was one of Mom's closest friends. They met in tap class. She also had ovarian cancer years before and had been in remission. When Mom was diagnosed, Judy was right by her side to talk her through everything. Judy even retained a port in her chest (where the chemo used to enter) as a good luck charm. She had a belief that as long as that port remained, she wouldn't get cancer again. However, her cancer did return, but this time in her mouth. Mom and Judy had supported one another and made a pact that they both would survive. It was a real blow to Mom's confidence when she found out about her friend's death.

When I spent the month of February with Mom, I went with the entire tap troop to see Savian Glover, one of the best-known tap dancers in the world. They had bought a row of tickets and invited Mom and Max as their special guests to celebrate all the work that she had put into the class. Mom was in the hospital, so I had the privilege of attending the show in her place. I took along one of my closest friends from college, Lea.

The show was absolutely amazing. At the end Lea looked at me and said: "We should go get Savian's autograph for your Mom."

"I doubt if we'll be able to do that," I said.

Lea's eyes went wide. "That does not sound like you. I've never heard you say something wasn't possible."

She was absolutely right. I guess I was so tired from the entire month of going through the surgery and being on edge about my mom's future, I wasn't myself. You know who your true friends are when they tell it to you straight.

I smiled at Lea. "Let's get it!"

Lea and I walked out of the theater and found the stage door down a flight of stairs. We knocked and knocked. No one came. At that moment, it was Mom's friend Judy whose tiny head appeared over the concrete wall and called down to us: "He's meeting with a group of kids in the lobby. There is a reception we can crash." I knew I liked Judy, and I appreciated her even more right then and there.

Lea and I ran back up the stairs. Sure enough there were drinks and food in the lobby and the entire Flamingo Ridge Tap troupe had made itself at home around a table. Savian entered the room and gave a speech to a group of aspiring, teenage dancers. As soon as he was free, Judy and Lea dragged me with them and we were at his side.

"Can you sign this program for my sister? She's in the hospital and couldn't make it tonight," Judy said. My heart caught in my throat. Mom and she had been like sisters—cancer sisters. They'd gone to chemotherapy together. They had talked about their lives, how they were feeling, and what they thought it would be like for their husbands if they died. Judy, like my mom, had red hair, and they had tapped together. How strange this cancer was; it created the most astounding relationships. Judy handed me the program so I could take it to my mom the next day in the hospital.

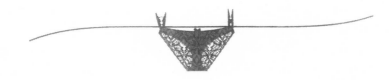

Chapter 39
A 10% Chance is
Better Than No Chance

I had stepped outside of Lucky Lu's Hair Salon to chat with Mom. I was pretty conspicuous there on the street corner outside even though I was trying my best to hide myself by facing the cement wall. My neighborhood was pretty small where folks knew each other and there I was in sunglasses, hair dye and foils on my head, a giant plastic bib around me. I didn't want to be on the phone. I didn't want to be having this call. I didn't want to hear the news that I knew was already coming. I was hyperventilating waiting for my mom to talk, trying to hold back the tears because I knew exactly what she was about to say and I hated life right then.

"Well, honey, we got the results and it isn't good. The cancer has been spreading so we can't continue with the trial."

I didn't say a word.

"Are you okay?" Mom asked.

"I am definitely not okay. I'm not okay at all. It isn't fair Mom. It isn't fair. It was supposed to work," I said balling my eyes out.

Mom let me be for a few minutes while I sobbed and tried to catch my breath. I hated myself for crying and putting more of a burden on her. I felt so trapped by Mom's diagnosis and by my own emotions. She was always the one I'd go to for comfort and I HAD to be strong for her. I willed myself to stop crying.

"I'll be okay Mom. What's next?" I asked her quietly.

"Well, Dr. S. says that there is one more type of chemo we can try and it has a 10% chance of working."

There is no way she should do it. She isn't going to do it is she? I thought to myself. But instead I calmly asked, "Are you going to try it?"

"We don't know. We just left the doctor's office. Max and I need to talk and figure that out."

"Well, you let me know what you decide. You know I'm okay with whatever you choose. Do you want me to come there and talk it through with you?"

"I know you'll support my decision, honey. Max and I will talk it over and we'll let you know."

"Okay Mom. I love you. Veeerrrry much," and hung up the phone.

I was stunned. I walked back in the salon and sat down in the chair. Lacey, the owner knew I had been waiting on the call. We'd been talking about it right before Mom called. I'd been crying and Lacey had just listened. She was such a cool chick.

She called herself a "hair slinger" and looked like tiny version of a pin up model from the 50's. She was drop dead gorgeous with this porcelain skin, ruby red lips and depending on her mood her hair could be fire engine red, blond bombshell or black as night. She decorated her salon in a retro '50s style – with 50's style barber chairs for us to sit in and antique vanities that she used for her two stations. She was magic with the scissors and every time I got a haircut from her, strangers stopped me on the street and asked where I got my hair done. She was that good.

Lacey took one look and me and I burst into tears as I sat down in her chair. I was trying so hard to hold it together but just couldn't. I shook my head and huge tears started rolling down my face. She gave me some tissues and started regaling me with stories about her son and her new boyfriend to take my mind off the situation.

I thought a lot about that conversation with my mom. I honestly couldn't fathom the fact that she had undergone this massive surgery and survived and that we had found this experimental drug she qualified for—all for nothing. I thought about everything my mom's poor body had been through. The surgery might have given her a few more months but she was in pain constantly, she couldn't eat the foods she liked, and she'd just undergone seven more rounds of chemo and lost all of her hair *again* and *it hadn't worked. Are you kidding me?*

"Where are you G-d? Life isn't supposed to go this way," I shouted at the ceiling of my bedroom later that night literally shaking my fist at the invisible G-d. I was furious, absolutely furious. I turned around and started beating my pillows with my fists and crying until I was exhausted. I'm sure my housemates heard me but they knew instinctively when to leave me alone and when to knock on my bedroom door and let themselves in.

What was Mom going to do? Her quality of life SUCKED right now. She could barely tap dance; she and Max couldn't really eat out any more either because she couldn't have most of what was on the menu. When they did eat out, she barely ate because, guess what sports fans? The tumor was now pressing in on her lungs and she could only get comfortable if she was reclined in a chair so restaurant chairs didn't do it for her. That meant that either Mom was getting the placebo or the experimental drug wasn't working on her – there really was no way to know. All we knew was that the cancer had continued to grow over the last seven weeks.

We should just get everyone together in Florida and have a celebration of her life I said to myself. She's had enough. Her body can't take it. Maybe if she was off of chemo she wouldn't be so weak and we'd have a month or two when she felt and looked a little better. We'll throw her an early birthday party and all of her friends will come and celebrate her. We won't wait for the funeral service. It would do Mom good to hear from her friends.

I hadn't heard from my mom in a few days so I called her.

"Mom I know we promised to say everything and to be truthful and honest right?" I was already crying.

"Yes honey," she responded.

"I don't think you should do this treatment. I think you've been through enough and we should get the family together and celebrate. That's what I think. Or if your doctors will let you, go on a cruise together and just be together. That's what I think," I finished.

When I finally stopped talking, Mom thanked me. She thanked me for saying everything. She thanked me for all of the suggestions. Then she said, "I'm not ready to go yet honey. I love my life too much to just give up even if it is only a 10% chance. I'm going to do the chemo. I'm not ready to leave Max. I'm not ready to leave you and the rest of the family. I'm just not ready to leave yet."

I sighed. My heart was heavy with grief because I knew death was so close and it expanded with love for my mom. I truly wasn't ready for her to go either but it wasn't up to me to keep her around. I wanted her to have the freedom to know that if she was tired and wanted to stop, she could. My ex-husband used to be an ICU nurse and he said the worst was when the patient was holding on for the family.

"Don't be like that Jen. Let her go on her terms. Don't be selfish and make her hold on for you," he had told me.

"You make a lot of sense Mom. So if you want to go for it, I'm behind you 100%."

"I knew you would be honey. You always are. Besides, my five-year cancer birthday isn't until August 10, so I've got to wait." We both chuckled and I was reminded once again of the horrific statistics Mom was handed upon diagnosis—less than an 18% chance of living five years or more. She had always said: "I'm going to be part of the 18%. Why not? Someone has to be." August 10 was the five-year anniversary.

I hung up the phone. A 10% chance. Okay. I'll take it. August 10 was still a few months away but I really wondered whether Mom would make it to my birthday on August 30.

"I am so selfish," I thought to myself.

Chapter 40
I Have No Bucket List

*M*om started the new chemotherapy regime. Unfortunately, the cancer continued to grow. By June of that year her CA-125 cancer marker was well over 600. Back in January, it had been at 18. After the marker results came in, the doctor sat with Mom and Max and told them that there was nothing more that she could do. The doctor was kind, as were all of her staff. She sat with my parents and cried with them a little. I could not imagine what type of person would choose oncology as a specialty when it was predictable that you would lose a large percentage of your patients.

"Jan, it's time for you to go and complete what is on your bucket list," she said with tears in her eyes.

I imagined Mom smiled compassionately not wanting to upset the doctor. Mom always worried about everyone else, right up to the end.

"I don't have a bucket list. I'm happy right here at home," was what Mom said.

Later on that morning Mom sent Aunt Jackie and me a note telling us what had transpired in the doctor's office. Now it was time for me to truly face the beginning of the end. This had been the most exhausting five years of my life, preparing for the end of my mom's life so many times. It was like riding a yo-yo or being on a roller coaster ride. I'd go into a visit with Mom thinking I needed to prepare for the end of her life, and then find hope and all the angst is erased. But only momentarily. It had been flat out exhausting in every way: mentally, emotionally, spiritually and physically. But in a weird way it was a good exhaustion because I really had, well, *we* really had left everything on the playing field. It was just like the quote from President Roosevelt that I had read long ago: "The credit belongs to the man who is actually in the arena, whose face is marred by dust and sweat and blood; who strives valiantly; who errs, who comes up short again and again..." We'd been in this arena for five long years.

I thought about what my mom wrote in her email: she didn't have a bucket list. She couldn't be totally satisfied with her life, could she? I mean doesn't everyone have those things on a list they want to achieve and hope to achieve once they get married, or the kids are gone, or they get their first job? Was she wholly satisfied with her life?

My mom raised my brother and me; she had a thirty-year career with the Federal Government; she had a thirty-year relationship with a man who loved her very much; she had four children, nine grandchildren and six great grandchildren; she had performed in plays and competed in tap dance shows. She returned to school in her fifties and received her PhD. She won awards. She had many friends who loved her. All this time, I imagined she longed for something more – things she had given up in sacrifice – and that somehow she was a victim of her life. But that wasn't the case at all.

My mother was satisfied with her life; satisfied with everything that had happened and accepting of everything that had not happened. If there was something she wanted to do, she would do it. If Max didn't want to join her, she didn't do it. That was okay because it was more important to her to have the man she loved with her when she did those things in her life that she cared about.

I thought about how brave my mother had been. When she and my father divorced when I was eleven, she was making $7,800 a year as a schoolteacher. My dad wasn't making much either and couldn't help out a lot. So Mom quit teaching and took a good paying job with the government that provided health care and retirement—a stability that was important to her because her kids were important to her. She never complained the way I imagined I would have. She chose that job. She chose to be divorced.

Once upon a time, she even kidnapped my grandmother from her job under the cover of night. My grandma had been working as head of housekeeping at a small resort in the Catskills. Mom and I stopped off to visit her on my way to camp and found Grandma, then in her seventies, scrubbing toilets. Apparently, the resort owners had run into financial problems and had to fire most of the staff. My grandma picked up the slack, never saying a word to us. Mom dropped me off at camp, returned with a U-Haul, and brought Grandma back to Ohio to live with us. It was a wonderful decision on my mom's part because now I had two strong female role models in the house.

As I thought a bit about my mom's life and how I thought it should be, I realized how few times I had chosen my life exactly the way it was and exactly the way it wasn't. When I was single, I wanted to be married. After a certain point in my marriage, I wanted to be single again. I was a consultant and wanted a full-time job. I got the full-time job and missed the flexibility of being a consultant. I moved to Colorado but missed my life in DC.

I had a bucket list filled with silly stuff. I imagined that most people had really serious, life-changing kinds of things like moving to India to live on an Ashram or discovering a new scientific theory. I also thought that most bucket lists have items that people are actually going to accomplish. Somehow the things on my bucket list were not things I thought I was ever going to accomplish. They were good ideas, whimsical ideas, flights of fancy, and things I might do someday but that I knew I wasn't going to do anything about. I wanted to cycle through Italy, I wanted to travel the world, and I wanted to see Neil Diamond in concert in Vegas with a bunch of friends dressed in terrible seventies clothes and arrive in a white stretch limo. I wanted to take an RV along Route 66 and take pictures and interview people I met along the way and write stories about it.

I wasn't doing anything about my list. My mother didn't have one. I never seemed to be satisfied with anything. Mom, on the other hand, was completely satisfied with her life exactly the way she had lived it. I had held the opinion that my mom had led a small life – that somehow she didn't get to do what she really wanted to do. How wrong I was. I was the one living a small life. I was the one dissatisfied. I was the one living a life constrained by walls of my own making.

Chapter 41
A Little Don Time

The day after Mom told me that she had been dropped from the experimental drug trial, I put my bike in the car and drove to my brother-in-law Don's house. Don and I had started a cycling group a few years back with my friend Lisa to ride the MS-150 together at the end of June. The ride was only a few weeks away and I knew I was in for a bit of a torture session because I had had little time to ride over the previous few months. We decided to do a 46-mile ride together. I was slower than Don, but he had a lot of patience and was happy to get the miles in even if it meant he rode more slowly than usual.

I was looking forward to spending time with Don. He was a great listener and a great coach. He had a very gentle and compassionate nature, which made him a terrific ICU nurse and father. It was more than that though. When you were around Don, there was no judgment. It didn't matter what you were dealing with or what mood you were in, Don always had a smile on his face and love in his heart for you. It was comforting to be in his presence.

"I need Don time," my ex-husband used to say to me. I could always tell when they had spent time together. Adam came back more reflective, relaxed and happier. Adam was there for Don when he needed him, too. They had lived together for a few years after Don's divorce. Don had been really down in the dumps and couldn't snap out of it. Adam, being a former mountain and road bike racer, bought Don a bike and they started riding together. Don gave Adam the credit for turning his life around at that point, so it was a mutual admiration society.

As usual, the sun was shining in Colorado—we had 333 days of sunshine a year. You couldn't beat it. Don lived near a few great trails that had rolling hills and beautiful views of the mountains. I was looking forward to my lungs straining to get air and my legs burning after not being on the bike for a while. Most people thought it was torture. I thought it was nirvana.

As we rode up the first hill, I noticed my breathing was off. I have sports induced asthma and always carry an inhaler, so I used it. As I watched Don disappear up the hill as if he were riding on a flat road, I struggled for breath. I knew he'd wait at the top. This went on for the first 15 miles or so. Don would shoot up hills and wait for me, or circle back to come get me. I just didn't feel right. My legs felt like lead. My lungs burned. I was using my inhaler much more than usual. On top of it all, I simply couldn't get comfortable in the saddle. What the heck was wrong with me?

"So, how's your Mom?" Don finally asked. We hadn't had much time to talk since I'd been such a slow poke. I filled Don in on the latest news. The doctor had sent Mom home because there was nothing more that she could do. Mom sent me an email a few days later to say that she and Max were heading up to Tampa to another cancer center to get a second opinion. Mom was looking into yet another alternative treatment. I just didn't understand why she was still searching for a cure. It was obvious to me what the outcome would be. Why keep trying when the predictable result would be the same. I was exhausted, wasn't she?

As I spoke, Don listened empathetically and asked questions from time to time. He had been a nurse working in the intensive care unit (ICU) and had a lot of experience dealing with death and with family members who were facing the death of their loved ones. We rode in silence for a while. Tears started forming at the corners of my eyes and slowly running down my face. I was hoping that Don wouldn't see. But I couldn't hold them back anymore. They came out with the fear, the exhaustion, the complete and total despair. I let out a strangled yelp and just started sobbing.

"I don't care about anything, Don. Mom is going to die. I mean I guess I knew that was going to happen at some point, but I haven't been able to fathom the reality. There is nothing more that we can do. I don't care about you, or this ride, or my job, or my friends, or anything, honestly. Is that normal? Is it normal not to care about any goddamn thing in the world? Mom's going to die and the world should stop, and it hasn't. How can the world just go on? How can I just ride a bike and pretend like it isn't happening? Why isn't the world stopping? She is going to die and I DON'T CARE ABOUT ANYTHING RIGHT NOW."

"Why don't we pull over and stop?" Don said quietly. At this point it had taken us nearly an hour to ride six miles, about a third of what we would usually cover in that amount of time. I realized why I had been struggling so very much with the ride that day. I didn't care.

We pulled over and Don held my bike while I shakily got off. He sat me down on a park bench and just held me while I cried for what seemed like hours. I had told my mom she would live. I had promised her that she would live. I had told her that I would do anything and everything in my power to make certain that she lived. And she was not going to live. I had failed.

I could not imagine a life without my mom. I couldn't imagine not being able to pick up the phone, or feel her arms around me, or hear her laugh.

"Is this normal?" I asked as my sobs finally started to subside.

"Of course it is," Don said softly. He told me it wasn't my fault and reminded me of a simple lesson: There are things we can't control in our lives.

Of course I knew all of this and had said them to others on many occasions. But it helped to hear these words from a friend. It was good to get out everything that was going on in my head so that I could stop thinking I was crazy.

"Honestly, Jen, I'd be worried if you were in any other place right now," Don said with his usual catching smile.

It dawned on me that Don was right. It would be weird. He gave me another hug, and we got back on our bikes, and we rode back to his house.

"Sorry you didn't even break a sweat," I told Don as I put my bike into the car and said goodbye.

"That's okay, this ride wasn't for me. It was for you." I had gotten my Don time and was more peaceful than I had been in months.

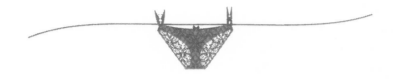

Chapter 42
That's Not Funny

All of a sudden it was August, and I was getting ready to spend a week celebrating my birthday with Mom and Max at the end of the month. In the back of my mind loomed the question: "Is this going to be the last time I will spend lucid time with Mom?" More than that, once she passed, what would my relationship with Max be? All these were questions I didn't know the answer to and didn't want to think about at that moment.

As the end of August approached, I was preparing to do a stand-up comedy showcase with my girlfriend Kristina Hall who had been a professional comic since the late eighties. She had been my mentor seven years before when I wanted to pursue my dream of performing stand-up comedy. She had appeared on more than 4,000 stages nationwide as well as on The Comedy Channel, Showtime and other television channels. She was brilliant and I was honored to open for her.

I had appeared on at least fifty stages in Colorado and one in Florida where I actually opened for an HBO comic and did a ten-minute set for an audience that had included Mom, Max and all of their friends from Flamingo Ridge. I had never been on TV but had participated in a showcase of Jewish comics for a nationally distributed Jewish magazine.

The show I was doing with Kristina was called "Hot Chicks with Brains." We figured if we weren't funny, at least there was truth in advertising (and we showed cleavage—always a plus). Our comedy was designed to stir the pot and get people talking about topics they didn't usually approach. No topic was too sensitive because Kristina had taught me to write about what was going in my life. Like any good comic, we found humor in every situation, no matter how tragic.

I had covered sex, dating, politics, religion and my divorce in previous performances. I generally drew upon exactly what I was dealing with at the time, but could I make jokes about Mom dying? Would my mom think it was funny? Would other people laugh? Or would they be horrified that I was making fun of someone whose life was about to end? I called Kristina and told her about my concerns. She reminded me that we were purposefully irreverent. "Get more committed to the difference you want to make with your comedy, Jen, than to what people will say. Who cares if they are offended? Offend them! Death is offensive." I got what she was saying and started writing.

I decided to call Mom and try out one of the jokes on her to see if she was okay with my writing about her cancer and impending death.

"Well, I don't know. Let me hear the joke, honey. Then I'll tell you," was all she said.

"Okay. Well remember the time that you told me you were going to get a second opinion? It's a joke based on that. Here's what I'm going to say. 'My mother has cancer, and her doctor of five years told her there was nothing more they could do. My mother decided to drive to Tampa to get a second opinion. I told her I could save her the time and gas money. 'How, honey?' she asked. I'll give you a second opinion Mom— you're dying!"

There was total silence. Oh crap, I thought, now I've done it. Then my mother burst out laughing and we laughed ourselves silly until we cried. "The funny part is that I did get a second opinion because, why not?" Mom told me to go ahead and use the material.

But the next day I received a phone call from her. "Honey, I thought about that joke and it really isn't funny." Uh oh, I thought.

"But do you want to know what is funny? Here's what is funny. When your Aunt Jackie was here we went shopping at St. Armand's Circle in this very exclusive store and I bought about $1,000 worth of clothes. I got them home and thought 'What am I doing? What if I die before I wear them? I'll leave the tags on so that Jennifer can return them and get the money back.' But today I decided screw it. I'm wearing the damn clothes, so all the tags are off. Too bad for you," Mom said, teasingly. We laughed until we cried one more time. It was wonderful that we could be so incredibly open and even laugh about what was going on.

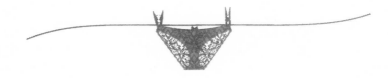

Chapter 43
Bring Out Your Thong

I was dreading arriving in August because I knew Mom's condition had deteriorated. She now hadn't had any chemo since the previous January and, as her doctor said, it was the chemo that had been keeping her alive all this time. When I landed at the airport I was surprised to see her in the front seat. She got out of the car to hug and kiss me. She looked beautiful as always, just rail thin and very tired.

She'd had a lot of company over the summer. Mom wanted to have special time with all of her kids. My brother Aaron had flown down around the Fourth of July weekend. He had just found a new job and it was difficult for him to take a lot of time off of work, so this was a really important visit for both of them. She was so very happy to see him and shared with me that if she didn't see him again before the end, it was would be okay. She loved him, and she knew he loved her and that was all that mattered.

Max's son Steve and his family came to visit in July. Max had two kids—Steve and Lisa. Steve and I were only a few months apart, as were Lisa and my brother Aaron. Steve was married to a wonderful woman named Beth who he had met in college and they had one son named Roger. I always called Roger "the cutest boy in the world." After I had sent him a birthday present when he was nine, I received a voice message: "Hello, hello, Aunt Jennifer? This is the cutest boy in the world—your nephew Roger." He was adorable. Lisa had eight children and five grandchildren. We never related to one another as "step" this or that— we loved each other and often saw each other during family vacations that Mom arranged. Sometimes it was a while between times we spoke, but that never mattered.

Steve and I were very close. I tried to fly to Minnesota at least once a year to spend some vacation time with him and his family. When they could, they came through Colorado to spend time with me. We had even camped together. I remember one visit; Steve was sitting by me while I opened up a birthday present he had gotten me. It was a Whoopee cushion! Steve and I kept blowing it up and making farting sounds, and we were crying from laughing so hard. Meanwhile, Beth was in the other room just chuckling and rolling her eyes at us. We all loved each other very much. It meant a lot to me that my stepsiblings, Steve and Lisa and their families, loved my mom so much.

So there I was in Florida with Mom for the week. We did all the things we loved to do. I went to tap class with her and, yes, she even got up to dance with the class. We ate out at her favorite restaurants. We had lunch with friends. Mom and I went shopping after one of those lunches and she bought two beautiful tops for me for my birthday. She sat in a chair and pointed at clothes she wanted me to try on. I remember my grandmother doing the same in her declining years and never complaining about being tired.

I noticed while I was there I seemed to be hypersensitive to Max and any comments he made to me or anyone else. I was disappointed in myself because I felt we truly had transformed our relationship that previous February. Things between us had been quite peaceful since that time. Something about this time was different. Perhaps we both knew it was the last time we'd all be together, and we were both on edge.

I did start to notice myself reacting each and every time an opinion about Max came up in my brain. However, I didn't give in to voicing the opinion. I didn't react. It was like I was in a movie theater watching my life. I watched as these two characters—Max and I—related to one another. I observed myself in the movie having opinions and judgments about Max and, instead of voicing them, setting them aside. I would recognize it as just an opinion and set it aside as that, and not the truth about Max. Each and every time I did this, my heart filled with love and compassion. Here was this man who had been married to my mother for more than thirty years, and he was watching her die before his eyes. He was helpless because there was nothing he could do about it.

As the week wore on, Mom and I talked about a lot of end-of-life issues. We met with a grief counselor to see if I had questions after reading the materials about hospice. She was astonished to hear Mom and I talking so openly—we even shared with her the jokes we had written. Mom showed me where the funeral home was, reminded me where the safe deposit box was, and where the important papers were.

We went through her jewelry box together so she could give me what she wanted me to have. We also went through her closet. Mom brought out special dresses and tops she wanted me to have.

"I want you to take my panties," she said deadpan.

"Excuse me?"

"I want you to take my panties. I have about 25 pairs of those Hanky Panky's—the ones I got you. They cost $20 a piece and I don't want them to go to waste."

Of course she didn't. She was one of the most budget conscious people I knew.

Besides, Hanky Panky's happen to be the most comfortable thong underwear a woman can wear. My mom actually turned me on to them years earlier and sent me half a dozen that she found on sale.

"You want me to take them now?"

"NO! I'm still wearing them."

"Mom! Mom! Why, oh why, did you have to tell me that," I said as I pounded the heel of my palm vigorously against my head trying to get the picture of her seventy-one-year-old butt in thong underwear out of my brain. Aargh. Seriously?

She laughed. "I just want to make certain that they don't go to waste. And remember *don't dry them.* They'll last longer."

She was always a logical planner. If it gave her peace of mind to know that I would wear the underwear, so be it. The conversations we were having were surreal. I suppose it was better this way, but I still felt like a vulture. Not only was the body still warm, the heart was beating.

"'Bring out your dead, I'm not dead yet, feel like getting up and walking around some! Feel like wearing my thong panties some,'" I giggled.

Mom looked at me blankly.

"It's a line from Monty Python's movie *Life of Brian,*" I said.

"They wore thong underwear in that movie?" she asked.

"Not exactly," I trailed off.

Of course my mom didn't get the line from Monty Python's *Life of Brian,* but I had to try. After all, this was the same woman who turned me on to the first episode of South Park where Jesus fights Santa Claus.

Chapter 44
The Most Beautiful
Birthday Card in the World

We spent the next few days taking care of some of the more mundane things around the house. We transferred the home phone, cell phone and utilities to Max's name. We wrote down all of Mom's passwords. We tried to show Max how to check his email. In fact, we tried a few times. He got impatient very quickly. He had not used the computer very much. He had relied on Mom for all things related to the computer. But my guess is that his impatience had little to do with what we were showing him. He simply couldn't or didn't want to cope with what was happening in the reality of the situation. As much as we knew these things had to be done, we found them excruciatingly painful to do.

On Sunday nights in Sarasota, people flock to Siesta Key Beach and watch the sunset together. People pour in from all over the area to form a drum circle. They drum together and dance to welcome the sunset. The tourists watch and clap with delight.

Mom had asked me to go with her several times, and I had always turned her down for one reason or another. On the one hand, I thought it was kind of cheesy. On the other, I thought I might go but simply figured we had plenty of time and would get to it. But now, Mom had run out of time. The last Sunday I was there in August I decided to go, alone, because she didn't have the strength to go with me. I was very sad. I had missed out going with her because I'd been too busy—with what I'll never remember. I was always on vacation when I was there. I just didn't make the effort. So I sat, I watched, I borrowed a drum, and I cried silently, tears rolling down my face, mostly sad with myself that I hadn't taken the time, once again, to do something Mom wanted us to do together.

I cried with regret. I cried because I felt guilty that I wasn't with her at home. I cried for all of the lost moments and memories. I also knew that if Mom knew I was feeling one bit of remorse, guilt or regret, she'd be angry with me. She didn't harbor any of those regrets. She just wanted me to be happy. Finally, as I watched the sky turn hues of orange-purplish-red, I took a few breaths and felt relief. Why waste another moment being upset? My mom wouldn't have.

I drove back to the condo to have dinner with Mom. She loved watching TV shows on BBC, and I loved watching her as she watched. Sometimes she laughed really hard and sometimes she'd cry. She wasn't laughing often these days, and I'd take every moment I could get. We sat in her office, she on her recliner so that her "cancer baby" didn't press into her diaphragm and, me on the loveseat across from her. At one point, she got up and left the room, only to return with gleeful eyes, holding up a bag of candy corn.

"The drugstore had them on sale. One dollar for the whole bag!" she exclaimed as she tore it open.

She settled into the recliner, put her feet up and sighed. I watched as she reached into the bag for a handful of the candy corn pieces, and then carefully rested them on the divot between her giant swollen belly and her breastbone.

"Mom, what are you doing?" I asked as she popped a piece in into her mouth.

She giggled. "I used to do this when I was pregnant with you."

"Eat candy off your pregnant belly?"

"No, I'd balance the ashtray on you so I could smoke a cigarette in one hand and drink my cocktail in the other," she laughed. "Every once in a while you'd kick the ashtray and we'd laugh and laugh," she went on to say.

"Mom!" I nearly choked. "I kicked because I didn't want you getting cancer!"

We laughed so hard we had tears streaming down our faces. Max came in to see what the commotion was but we couldn't breathe so we couldn't tell him what was going on. He just waved his hand at us and said, "You two," and went back into the living room. That made us laugh even harder.

My trip was over and it was time for me to leave. As we drove to the airport at the end of the trip, my eyes welled up with tears. I didn't want to think about the next time I'd be in Sarasota because I knew without a doubt it would be to be with Mom as she received hospice care. I turned my head to look out the window so she couldn't see me crying. I wiped away the few tears that trickled down my cheek as quickly as possible and sighed.

"You okay, honey?" my mom asked.

"Yeah, Mom. I'm fine," I said without my voice cracking, miraculously.

Mom turned around to smile at me and hand me a birthday card. I opened the envelope and inside was the most beautiful card I had ever seen. Not only was it visually stunning, but the message itself also blew me away. It talked about how proud they were of me as their daughter, how much they cherished me, and how successful they knew I'd be.

I stared down at the card—at Mom's and Max's signatures. This would be the very last time I'd see her signature on a card. It would be the last time I received a card like this, so mushy and heartfelt. It just wasn't Max's way. This was a Mom kind of card.

"You know, Max picked out that card," Mom said as she turned to me and smiled.

My heart caught in my throat. Max picked out the card? Wow, I didn't know Max at all. I was so quick to judge—just another opinion among the sea of opinions rattling around in my brain. I was so glad I had kept putting aside those opinions all week so I could truly see the depth of Max's love.

I got out of the car and hugged Mom tightly as I said goodbye. She felt so small and frail, I was afraid I would crush her. Then I turned to Max for a hug. "Goodbye Jennifer," he said. "Thanks for coming." This was the usual cue to let go, so I did. But for the first time in 30 years, Max didn't let go first. He held on. So did I. Had I held on to my judgments and opinions, I wondered what the outcome would have been. I wouldn't have been so open with my love and might have missed this warm embrace. When we eventually let go, we both had tears in our eyes.

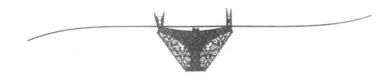

Chapter 45
My Whole Heart
Rises Up in Thankfulness

*I*n September, Aunt Jackie and Uncle Joe flew down to see Mom. Uncle Joe is petrified of flying but wanted to make the trip because he suspected it would be one of the last times he would see my mom. Seeing my Uncle Joe and Max together was hilarious—the two of them just giggled and laughed and made fun of each other. Max needed to laugh.

My Aunt Jackie and my mom, on first glance, were so very different. Mom was pale with red hair and freckles that she inherited from her mother. My aunt had an olive complexion, dark brown eyes, and hair that definitely took after the Italian side of the family.

The three of us had been together back in Cleveland, one time, visiting my grandmother in the hospital. Aunt Jackie had asked for the car windows to be opened so we could get some fresh air, but Mom didn't want the breeze to blow her hair out of place. An hour later Jackie and I stepped out to get some lunch. As soon as we got into the car, we looked at each other and rolled down the windows to enjoy the wind in our hair after being cooped up in the hospital all morning.

That was typical, really. Jackie could go with the flow and Mom liked plans and structure.

Even with their differences, they forged a special sisterly relationship that just got stronger after Mom got sick. They would chat on instant message while Mom was getting chemo. The three of us took on emailing every day or so to stay caught up on what we were doing. I got to know Aunt Jackie and Uncle Joe a lot better over those last few years.

Jackie and Joe were staying next door in Sarasota, and one evening around eleven p.m., they heard a knock at the door. It was Max. He asked them to get dressed and come over to talk with him and Mom. Mom had signed up for hospice in the middle of August. "Just in case you need it," her doctor had said. She was glad she did because there were a few times that a night nurse had to come help her with her pain and digestive issues.

As predicted after the last surgery and without the help of chemo, the cancer was beginning to block her intestines once again. Mom and Max felt it was time to get her to hospice. She wasn't keeping food down normally and she couldn't control the pain. They wanted Jackie and Joe's input. The four of them sat around the dining room table, cried and made arrangements for Mom to go to hospice in the morning.

Mom and Jackie obviously spent a lot of time discussing practical matters that night. The immediate family received this email from Jackie on September 7.

Good Morning family,

As you know, Joe and I were in FL this past week, visiting with Jan and Max. I'm attaching a photo of the four of us at dinner at Stoneybrook on September 2. Although I love having blinders on, I know it's not real life and I need to face the near future with realism. (I still hope the "near" future is not so near, and that it is filled with comfort and love for both Jan and Max.)

Jan is adamant about people dressing informally at the service. She does not want ties, suits, jackets, etc. She told me that it shouldn't be a "private" service, i.e., invitation only. Anyone who wants to attend is welcome. And she told me to bring scissors in case any one does show up in a tie.

At Jan's request, we'll have a little reception after the service to celebrate Jan's life. If you have any questions, suggestions, or just want to talk, Joe and I are available via email or phone. Let's send Jan the most powerful vibes and prayers for a "beautiful death."

In the mean time I had been interviewing for a new job in Washington, DC and was scheduled to go for a final, in-person interview on September 8. I had shared my mom's condition and the uncertainty of how things would unfold with my future employer. I asked my mom if I should hold off on the interview and come stay with her in hospice instead. "Nope honey, you go for your interview," was her reply.

As I sat in the Denver airport waiting for my flight to leave for DC, I received a phone call from Mom.

"Honey, I'm writing an email to send to friends. I want them to know what is happening. Can I read it to you?" she asked.

"Of course you can," I replied.

I sat and listened to the email—it was sweet and poignant, but optimistic and practical all at the same time.

"Mom, I have only one addition. Let people know that you may not respond to their emails or phone calls. You don't need that added pressure right now."

"You are right honey, I'll add that line and send it out," she replied.

"Mom, I don't have to go for this interview. It can wait. I can come now. I can change my plane ticket," I said as I started crying.

"Is that for you or for me?" she asked. "Because I will tell you when I need you, and I don't need you now, okay? You go for your interview. That is where you need to be," she replied.

I smiled through my tears. My mom was still there, even as sick as she was—headstrong and stubborn, loving and beautiful. She was right. Flying to be with her was for me. I thanked her for always doing things her way. I hung up the phone and tears rolled down my cheeks as I sat waiting for my plane. I sincerely hoped, as Mom did, that she'd be a hospice miracle. Most people who check into hospice die within twelve days. She wanted to check out under her own steam. I never contradicted her because it had been her indomitable spirit that had kept her alive all this time.

I checked into my hotel room that evening and found this email from her in my inbox:

Hi, Dear Family and Friends,

I'm writing to you all at once to give you the latest update on my health. As you know, things haven't been great these past six months.

Still, the Energizer Bunny has kept going. At the encouragement of my oncologist when we started the anti-estrogen pill, I signed up with hospice, although at the time I wasn't in need of their services.

Her thought was that they'd have baseline on my 'new-normal' and would be immediately available when I did need them. After a few days, I did sign up.

When my pain increased, the additional narcotics caused other problems. I was glad I had signed up with hospice because I needed to call them twice after 9 p.m. A nurse also made a house call at two different evening times.

Unable to resolve the problem at home, I came to a hospice house for a few days for evaluation and pain management. So far the best combination has been IV drugs. Don't know when/if I'll be going home so I can't give you a prognosis. If going home is not an option without nursing care, we'll put in a request for a transfer to Sarasota where no beds were available at the time I entered or we'll make at-home arrangements. Stay tuned.

I welcome your emails. Know that I will read them all, although I may not respond. I prefer email to phone calls. Meanwhile, know that I'm grateful to have had you in my life and thank you for the gifts of caring, sharing, and love over the years.

To be sure this reaches everyone, especially those without email, please feel free to pass on the information.

Love, Jan

> *My whole heart rises up in thankfulness.*
> **—Robert Browning**

I read the email and marveled at my mother's ability to stay focused on others during such times of pain. I don't know if I would be as capable of being so selfless. I sincerely hoped I would. I landed in DC, had my interview, and was back in Colorado the evening of the eighth.

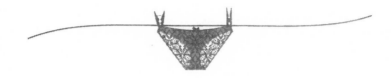

Chapter 46
It's Time

It was the start of Labor Day Weekend and friends from Los Angeles were arriving. They had made a documentary film about climate change and were traveling the country showcasing the film and drumming up support. They were driving a renewable energy bus, and my house had enough space out front for them to park the bus and sleep downstairs in sleeping bags. I couldn't wait to see my friend Michael. He was an actor from LA and had always impressed me with his wit and heart. We had gotten to know each other well over the years.

I stayed in touch with my mom, Max, my siblings, my aunt and uncle throughout the weekend. Michael and I spent many hours talking about what he was currently dealing with in his marriage, and my thoughts and feelings about my mom.

On Sunday, I joined the merry cast of characters and drove over to a local park for outdoor yoga. Imagine three hundred yoga enthusiasts spending two hours with a charismatic yogi under a bright blue sky near a manmade lake. It was exactly what I needed to let go of all of the stress that I had been carrying around for so long. We were tired and sweaty afterwards, but I felt balanced and centered.

We walked back to the bus to towel off and pass out flyers for the next showing of the documentary film. I turned on my phone and saw I had a message. People had been flocking to the bus since the yogi announced what Michael and his crew were up to, so I stepped away to get some quiet.

I was standing near a giant oak tree. As I listened to the message, my knees buckled. It was Max's voice—he was trying to hold it together on the phone but couldn't.

"Jennifer, your mom wanted me to call. It's time. It's time for you to come," he said through his tears.

I stumbled backward and put out my hand to steady myself against the giant oak. I slid down the tree to sit, uncontrollably sobbing, shaking, and wailing. Michael came running over and took me in his arms. I sat with him holding me for what felt like an hour. He said nothing. He didn't console me. He didn't have to say anything because there was nothing he could say that would make it okay. He did what was right and necessary—he just let me be. He just let me be sad.

When I finally calmed down he asked what was going on and I told him. He helped me call the airlines and book a ticket for the next day. Then we took the bus to a health food store and shopped for a really healthy and nutritious dinner. "You need nutrients," he kept saying to me. He picked out some healthy snacks for the plane. "You're dehydrated from yoga and all of that crying," he said as he put coconut water into the cart.

We got home, he made dinner and then helped me pack. We sat together watching the sunset over the mountains and I just cried and cried. Again, he said nothing and let me be. He just let me be with all of the sadness, the grief, and despair. His colleagues were just as gracious and loving. I kept telling him over and over again how important it was that he was there and how there were no accidents. He was the perfect person for me to be with in those moments. He didn't give me platitudes like, "Everything is going to be okay" or "Time heals all wounds." He just let me be without adding anything and without changing what I was going through. This was the best gift he could have given me.

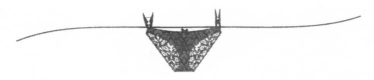

Chapter 47
Hold On

The next day I flew into Sarasota. Max picked me up from the airport. We had little to say to each other. We simply held hands in the car. Mom was being transported from a hospice facility a few hours from the house to one that was only twenty minutes away. We drove over there to meet her.

I walked into the room that she would occupy, for how long I had no idea. The room was filled with hotel style furniture with a big hospital bed in the middle. It could have seemed sterile, but it wasn't. There was a veranda and, beyond that, a butterfly garden. I was glad my mom would be able to look out the window and enjoy the flowers and the butterflies.

I sat on the couch nervously awaiting her arrival. What would she look like? Could she look any worse than she did last time? To be clear, Mom never looked "bad." She was always smiling—whether she had makeup on or not. Honestly, my mom didn't need makeup, but she thought she did. She just looked very skinny, and each time I saw her she appeared thinner and thinner. My phone rang.

"Hi Mom," I said.

"Hi honey, where are you?"

"I'm at the hospice center waiting for you, Mom," I replied.

"Oh good, we're just pulling in now. I'm so excited to see you."

I choked back a sob once again. "I'm excited to see you too, Mamasan."

About ten minutes later she was wheeled into the hospice room. She gave me a big smile and a wave and motioned me over to give me a hug before the nurse had stopped the chair. She asked about my flight and how I was able to get such a cheap ticket. I told her that the airline was absolutely amazing and how the person on the phone had worked with me to get the ticket last minute.

My mother was always very particular about things. She liked things just so. We spent the next half hour unpacking her belongings, setting up her music, hooking up her computer, and putting her lip balm and glasses within reach.

We spent some time together talking about nothing of any significance or importance. The doctor on duty came in to talk to Mom and ask her what her goals were in coming to hospice.

"Well, we're managing the pain. So ultimately, I'd like to go home if that is an option. If not, I'd like to be as comfortable as possible." I marveled at Mom's calm demeanor.

The doctor left and Max went back home to call his kids to find out when they were planning to come see Mom.

"Only if it works for them. You know that, don't you, love?" she called after Max as he walked out the door. Of course he knew that. My mom never wanted to put anyone out.

Finally, we were alone. I had a burning question I'd wanted to ask her for quite some time. The first four years of her cancer were easy, if that word can be used to describe anyone's terminal illness. But since the surgery in February, this year had been really rough. Her quality of life hadn't been good although she never missed her Tuesday tap class.

"Mom, I've been wondering. Are you sorry that you had the surgery last February? This year has been so hard on you and Max."

She looked at me and thought about my question carefully.

"I don't regret the surgery. I wasn't ready to go yet. While I didn't have all the mobility I would've liked, I wanted more time."

I felt relief course through me. I knew it had been her decision to have the surgery, and hers alone. I had been wondering whether our conversation in the ER had influenced her to do something she honestly didn't want to do. As much as I had stood for supporting her choices, I had been feeling guilty but now I could let that go.

Monday turned into Tuesday, and Tuesday turned into Wednesday. The three of us spent time together reading the paper, listening to music, and taking care of last minute paperwork that Max was worried about. We didn't know the prognosis of Mom's disease, but Mom, ever positive, told the doctor her intention was to return home.

My brother Steve arrived on Wednesday. Aaron was arriving on Friday and Lisa couldn't get to us until Sunday because she was observing the Sabbath and couldn't fly until then.

Steve, Max and I met with the hospice nurse and doctor to discuss Mom's condition. Mom had a morphine drip, but she also had a pain button to press to increase the dosage when she needed it. The doctors kept track of the extra pumps and kept increasing the IV medication accordingly.

I called my friend Esther who had been a hospice nurse for many years and filled her in on everything going on. She assured me that the purpose of hospice was to ensure that Mom wasn't in pain and to let the nurses do their job. While I trusted the hospice nurses who were working, it was nice to be reassured by a trusted friend.

Thursday wasn't a good day for Mom. She slipped in and out of sleep. The three of us would excuse ourselves to go cry or walk the grounds. We were pretty certain that Mom might pass that evening, but none of us wanted to actually say that.

I went for a run on the beach and Steve was able to take Mom in her wheel chair out to see the butterfly garden. She seemed to enjoy her outing. Mom also spoke to Lisa and reassured her that it was okay that she couldn't be there until Sunday.

As we left that night I hugged her. I whispered in her ear, "Mom, hold on for Aaron, he's coming tomorrow." She whispered back "I'll hold on for him, but I can't wait for Sunday for Lisa." I had spoken to Lisa and she understood that Mom might not be able to hold on that long. I reassured Mom that was okay and that Lisa understood.

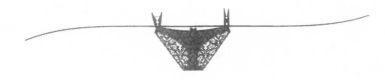

Chapter 48
Time Is an Illusion

The next morning instead of going straight over to hospice, I went to a much needed yoga class and treated myself to a leisurely breakfast with a friend.

Max and Steve were taking the morning shift so I could head back to the house and get Aaron's room ready for him. As I was driving there, Max called me. "You'll never believe who called me this morning? Jan Storti herself. Just like she was right here. I thought we were going to lose her last night, but she called and sounded so very strong." Max's voice broke as he blew his noise.

I started crying. I couldn't believe it. As Max was telling me this news, my mom beeped through. "Max, that's Mom calling. Let me take her call."

"Hi, Mom. How are you?" I asked with a slight smile on my face, holding my breath to see how she was doing.

"I'm good honey. Where are you? What are you doing?" she asked. She spoke as if she wasn't in hospice at all. Her speech was clear and unaffected by the drugs I knew she was on.

"Well, I just came from yoga class, and I'm heading home to get the room ready for Aaron," I told her.

"Oh that's right. You said you were going to yoga. Wait a minute. Aaron is coming? That's great," she sounded so happy.

I breathed a sigh of relief. She had heard me ask her to hold on for Aaron.

Mom sounded lonely, so I asked if she wanted me to come right over and help her with her hair and makeup. She said yes, so I called Max and told him I was taking the morning shift. As I walked in, the night nurse stopped me. She was a resident of Flamingo Ridge and knew my folks. She told me that my mom had seemed lonely the night before and that morning and that is why she had called us so very early. "She's been up since six-thirty. You might want to think about staying over tonight for her," she told me.

I walked into Mom's room and she was already up and dressed, with full make-up and wig. She was sitting on the couch with her computer propped on her lap and reading emails.

"Hi, honey. Come sit next to me and read all of these nice emails that people sent back in response to the email update on September 8th. I can't believe what people are saying about me. I guess this is what you wanted me to hear when you talked about having a life celebration," she said.

I told her it was exactly what I wanted her to hear. I wanted her to know, in her bones, the difference that she had made with each and every person in her life. She wanted to respond but said she was too tired. She was glad that we had specifically stated in the emails that she might not respond at all. "I don't want to disappoint anyone."

Mom closed her computer and set it aside. She looked at me and smiled as she picked up the scarf she was crocheting for my sister-in-law, Beth. She had made a scarf for each of us, as well as for some of her closest friends at Flamingo Ridge. As I watched her use her crochet hook, I became very sad. I'd never had another moment to ask her to teach me what she was doing. I had always been too busy to learn. Busy with what, I didn't remember.

Before each visit with Mom, we'd had a list of things we wanted to do—make a scrapbook, clean out closets, and teach me to crochet. Over the past year, I'd made sure some of those things got done that she could no longer do, like cleaning or sorting paperwork to get ready to transfer accounts to Max. But honestly, most of the time I was too busy with work and would get caught up in making phone calls or checking emails. I sighed deeply and tears formed in my eyes.

I looked at my mom. She held up the crochet hook very close to her eyes. She was swaying a bit back and forth while seated, attempting to focus through her morphine haze. She was sitting straight up on the couch and I knew it was uncomfortable because the tumor was pressing into her diaphragm. I didn't want to offer to help right away because sometimes she would get upset that I didn't think she could do something on her own. So I waited.

Finally, she put the hook down and sighed deeply. Tears formed in her eyes. "Can I help?" I asked. "I guess you can," she replied. I gently took the hook from her hand, as she sat back on the couch. She breathed deeply. "That's better," she said. She seemed so very small and defeated.

"What do I do Mom?" I asked. "You want to close off the end of the scarf, otherwise it will unravel," she explained. "I don't know what I'm doing though," I said. "I don't either honey, just do the best you can," she said.

So I sat with the crochet hook, and painstakingly finished the scarf, doing the best I could, just like my mom asked me to. She sat next to me with her eyes closed. I thought of all those times I had been too busy to learn from her as an adult. I thought about her teaching me macramé as a child and the hours of fun we had had making belts and jewelry. I had time then. But as an adult, somehow, I didn't have enough time or thought I'd have plenty of time to do these things later. I shook my head. Time truly is an illusion.

When I was done, I held it up to her. "How does that look?" I asked. "It's beautiful honey," she said trying to focus. "Can you get me back in bed. I'm tired."

I bent over to let Mom grip my forearms and pull herself up. I was afraid to take her arms. They were so birdlike. I thought I would break them or tear her skin. I walked her gingerly over to the bed and helped her in, straightening her bedclothes and arranging her table just so—phone within reach, glasses within reach, lip balm up on its end, and tissues nearby. She lay back and sighed as she closed her eyes. "I'm going to take a little nap."

I sat on the couch in Mom's hospice room in a state of disbelief. Not denial, because it was clear she had hours or maybe a few days left. In disbelief that her death was actually going to happen, I truly hoped she would hold out until Aaron arrived. I sat on the couch, one eye on the butterfly garden, the other eye on my mom, watching her breathe.

I must have dozed off too, because next thing I knew Max and his son were there, with Aaron bringing up the rear. Mom woke up and smiled a warm greeting as soon as they walked in the room. They encircled her bed. Max leaned over and gave Mom a kiss: "Hello Storti.

Guess who's here," he said, pointing to Aaron. Mom struggled to focus on Max, moved her head slowly toward his son Steve, and then zeroed in on my brother Aaron.

Her eyes popped open, she perked up and broke into the biggest grin I'd seen since arriving. She grabbed him by his goatee, and just stared at him. Aaron, seemingly unfazed by her appearance, simply said: "You like that, huh?" and chortled. They stared into each other's eyes for what seemed like a long time. He and Mom had a very special bond, and she loved him unconditionally. Her face said it all.

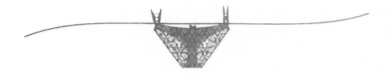

Chapter 49
I Wonder

Soon after Aaron arrived, I returned home to change the sheets on the bed and move my things over to Teri's house. As usual her door was open and my bedroom was awaiting my arrival. I took some time to sit on her loveseat overlooking the bay. I stared out at the sunshine and thought about my mom's relationship with my brother. Truth is I was jealous.

I knew in my bones that Mom loved me unconditionally but how on earth could she love him the same? He wasn't around like I was. He didn't call as often as I did. He didn't participate in family gatherings—it wasn't his style. I was always there, the responsible one, the good daughter.

I hated myself for having all of these thoughts. I hated that I was jealous. I hated myself for judging him and Mom's love for him. I hated that I didn't have the kind of relationship with him that I fantasized about—the kind where I could just collapse into his arms and cry about how sad I was going to be when Mom died. I hated myself for all the times I had tried and failed to be the kind of sister I thought he wanted me to be. I hated that I thought there was a kind of sister I should be. I hated that I had conditions on our relationship. I hated him for a minute. I hated myself for a minute. For a brief moment I even hated my mom. I hated that I hated.

As I sat there watching the birds soar across the sky and listening to the lapping of the waves against the mangrove trees, an idea bloomed in my head. The thoughts I was having weren't new. I'd had them plenty of times before. What if those thoughts were simply based on everything I thought I already knew about Aaron? On everything I thought I already knew about me? On everything I thought I already knew about my mom? On how I thought relationships "should be" between brothers and sisters? What if I didn't know anything at all? What if I didn't know my brother? What if we had no past relationship, or there were no ideas of how things "should be" in my head? I sat and stared at the water and let go of all of those opinions and began to wonder about my relationship with Aaron.

I felt my heart expand and my chest get warm. I recognized in that moment that my brother is my brother and I'll never have another one. I realized that I didn't know him and that anything I did know was based on a teenager's perspective, given that we hadn't spent a lot of time around each other over the last thirty years or so. I hadn't reached out to him very much. I hadn't loved him unconditionally but expected him to love me that way. I realized that my mother had it right all along—love unconditionally, give everything, and expect nothing in return.

My love was conditional, not just with my brother, but with lots of people. My ex-husband's face flashed before my eyes, as did the faces of other friends and family members. I let out a great long sigh, and allowed myself to get present to what I might have missed. Then, I forgave myself for what I did and for what I didn't do. In that moment I loved myself unconditionally and what became possible for me was to love everyone else unconditionally, as well.

I began to wonder about this talented musician and computer genius we called Aaron. I wondered about who he was, what his life was about and what it might be like for him to lose his mother. I had never even bothered to ask him how he was doing and what his world was like. I was only interested in him getting mine. I vowed to bring wonder to our relationship, to love him unconditionally, and to be truly interested in his world for the first time in my life.

It's funny. With anyone else in my life I would've come clean and told them what I had realized. But I didn't do that with my brother. He was a man of action, not words. He didn't talk a lot and he definitely never spoke about his feelings. Even when we had gotten into fights before and I attempted to apologize, he'd look at me with a blank stare and say: "I have no idea what you are talking about." In this case, actions were going to speak louder than words.

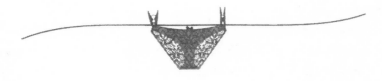

Chapter 50
A Sleepover

I drove back to hospice later that day. I entered the room and leaned over to give Mom a kiss and a hug. She was sitting in a reclining chair in the corner of the room. I could see Aaron outside near the butterfly garden, pacing and smoking. G-d, what I would have given to smoke a cigarette right then. Max and Steve were on the couch to my left, looking at Mom's computer. I sat down on the loveseat next to them.

"Well, we were just discussing whether Storti would like company tonight, but Storti won't tell us yes or no," Max said to me.

"Jan, would you like one of us to stay over tonight?" my stepbrother Steve asked.

Mom didn't answer. She just smiled.

"I don't know right now," she finally managed.

We had been increasing her morphine daily, based on the doctor's recommendation. As he had explained, Mom could increase the morphine by pushing a button. He would then increase her drip according to the number of times she hit the button over the course of a few hours. Each time they consulted the family to ensure it was what we wanted. We always agreed with the increase.

I remembered seeing the night nurse that morning, the one who knew her from Flamingo Ridge. She told me how the small loveseat in Mom's room could open out into a bed. I told her I'd discuss it with Max and Mom because I wanted my mom to have a say in every step of her treatment for as long as she could. If she didn't want someone to stay over and wanted privacy, then we wouldn't stay over.

I also wasn't certain if she would want Max or me. I was scared that if I did stay over and she died in the middle of the night, she might come to me like an apparition from Fiddler on the Roof—all white-faced and scary. I recalled a roommate in college recounting the time she was with her brother when he died. She told me that a person's last breaths were the hardest to hear. "They call it a death rattle for a reason," she had told me. Well, I guessed I would deal with that when it happened, I told myself.

Max, Aaron and Steve had left to go get lunch and have some downtime. I had a newspaper with me, so I began to read it while Mom dozed in her chair. After a while, I noticed that she was awake.

"Hi, Mommy," I said smiling at her. I wanted to broach the topic of someone staying over that night without the guys in the room.

"So, what do you think about Max's question? Do you want one of us to stay over with you? I'll do whatever you want, Mom," I said. I knew she had heard me, but she was silent for a long time. She was looking down at her hands. I wasn't sure how much she could comprehend. I took a breath and waited.

She nodded her head. "Yes, I would like someone to stay over. It was lonely this morning," she said.

"Do you want me or Max to stay over? I'm happy to stay, but if you'd rather have Max, just say the word. Whatever you want, Mom."

"I want you to stay over, honey, you seem to have the most patience," she said.

I smiled. "Okay, Mom. Whatever you want."

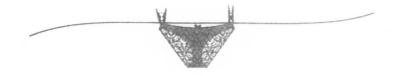

Chapter 51

Fred Astaire and
Ginger Rogers

I called Max and Steve and told them that Mom wanted me to stay over. They would bring me clothes when they came for dinner. Later that evening, the nurses helped me pull out the loveseat and put the sheets and small blanket on the bed. Once they had settled Mom down, I reached up to turn off the light.

"If you need anything, Mom, I'll be right here," I said.

"You always are, honey," she replied.

I turned out the light and pulled my eye-mask over my eyes. There was an eerie glow to the room because there were fluorescent lights that stayed on throughout the night. I hoped that Mom and I would be getting a good night's sleep but mostly I hoped she wouldn't die in the middle of the night.

I had barely shut my eyes when I heard Mom trying to get up from the bed. I yanked off the eye mask, leapt out of bed and positioned myself directly in front of her. At this point, she was so wobbly from the morphine she couldn't even lift herself out of bed. But she hated me pulling her up because she hurt everywhere so I just stretched out my arms so that she could grab hold and pull herself up at her own pace. Her pupils were so dilated that I couldn't distinguish between her pupil and her iris. It was like staring into two black marbles. She smiled at me and made kissing motions with her lips. I leaned over to kiss her. As I leaned over she pulled me into an unsteady embrace, and began scratching my back—her signal for me to scratch hers. I reached behind and as delicately as I could, scratched her back, my fingers scraping against every vertebra.

I took a deep breath and started sobbing in her arms. "Mom, I love you so very much, and I am going to miss you so very much," I whispered in her ear, finally understanding what she had been getting at the previous February in the emergency room when she said she would miss "this"—the actual physical connection. I would miss it too – the ability to reach out and hug her and smell her perfume and feel her arms around me. I cried in her arms as she held me and told her I loved her. As I pulled away she looked deep into my eyes, her own eyes filled with tears. She made kissing motions with her mouth, and I leaned over to kiss her again. I knew she knew I had finally understood her point.

I walked backwards with her holding my arms to take her to the bathroom—my Ginger Rogers to her Fred Astaire—until I turned her around so she could sit down on the toilet. I gently moved her IV out of the way as she gripped the grab-bar and lowered herself down. I reached to help her wipe herself and she shooed me away. "I can do it myself," she said. She then walked herself over to the sink to wash her hands and back into bed she went. The entire dance took about ten minutes from start to finish. It was eleven p.m.

We danced together in this way nearly every 30 minutes for the rest of the evening into sunrise. Mom said she was worried about how much sleep I was getting. I told her I was fine. Really, I was exhausted: exhausted from watching her struggle throughout the night to only get relief for a few moments; exhausted from telling her everything was going to be okay when I knew it wasn't; exhausted from keeping my own emotions in check so that I wouldn't upset her more. When six a.m. hit, we turned on the television and watched a ballet. I dozed on and off dreaming about Fred and Ginger until the nurses came in to bring her something to eat.

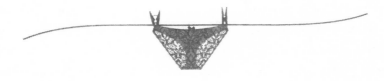

Chapter 52

If You Can't Pee, I Won't Pee

That morning Steve brought me breakfast and a change of clothes, and we sat with Mom until Max and Aaron arrived. The head nurse wanted to speak with us about next steps for Mom because had been quite agitated since she woke up that morning. She couldn't get comfortable and continued to need to get up to urinate at least every 30 minutes. Once there, only a few drops would pass from her bladder. I knew she was getting weaker and weaker. After a while I began to wipe her and wash her hands for her — it broke my heart to see her so incapacitated.

After consulting with the nurses, we agreed to give Mom a catheter and some anti-anxiety medication to help her sleep. While the nurses didn't exactly say this, we knew they were doing their job of making her as comfortable as possible because her time was close. I remember looking down at the catheter bag next to Mom's bed and being shocked that there were twenty ounces of urine in it. Twenty ounces? They had just put the catheter in less than an hour before. That was just over a half a quart of urine that had been in her bladder. The cancer was really blocking her ability to pass things out of her system. Ouch.

Aaron had to take a plane home early the next morning. He sat with Mom and arranged her pillows for her so that she was as comfortable as she could possibly be until it was time for him to go. I don't recall whether Mom was alert when Aaron left. I imagined it must have been difficult for him to leave, knowing that the next time we were together would be for her funeral. The question was how soon?

Max chose to stay over with me that evening. I asked him if he wanted to be by himself, but he assured me it was fine I was there. By this point Mom was only waking up every few hours or so but only briefly. We had a moment to say goodnight to her and tell her we loved her. I was grateful for Max's company and for knowing that I would actually get some sleep that night. Or so I thought.

Max slept on the leather lazy boy recliner, and it made noise every single time he moved. He was restless from the moment I laid my head down. I heard him get up and down quite a few times in the middle of the night until it seemed he was going to the bathroom as often as Mom had the night before. Thankfully Mom hadn't been awakened by Max's frequent trips to the bathroom. Neither did she wake up as we left to get Max to the emergency room to be treated for a urinary tract infection at six-thirty that next morning!

From the waiting room, I called Steve, Aunt Jackie and Uncle Joe to tell them the news. I sat there shaking my head from side to side.

Seriously? I had heard of men gaining pregnancy weight but this? What next? If only Mom knew this was happening, she would have had a good laugh. It was as if Max took on the infection that Mom should have had, given how long she'd been unable to pass urine out of her system. By 10:00am, I was dropping Max off at home. Steve was there to care for that patient and I would return to hospice to be with Mom later that day and after I worked out and changed my clothes.

Chapter 53
No One's Home

I was truly exhausted when I walked into Teri's condo around ten-fifteen but I knew I wouldn't be able to sleep. I was a morning person and it really never mattered what time I went to sleep because by seven a.m. or so I was always wide-awake. I sat with Teri and gave her an update, had some coffee, changed into my running clothes, and headed for Siesta Key Beach.

I wasn't supposed to run—doctor's orders, I had always explained. I had no cartilage under my right knee and had had knee surgery a few years before. A well-known sports medicine specialist in Colorado had advised me that if I wanted to keep cycling, I needed to give up running. Today, I was not going to listen to him because I knew I needed to expel all of the pent-up energy and frustration from the past week.

Siesta Key Beach is the most beautiful beach in the world. As the travel books say, "World's finest, whitest sand." The beach is made up of million-year-old quartz crystals pulverized to a fine white powder. Even on the hottest of days, the sand is cool to the touch. It makes it the perfect place to run barefoot, which is what I did. I needed to connect with the earth, feel the sand between my toes, and be able to run in and out of the water.

I started out with a slow jog, turning my face up to the sun and welcoming its heat piercing the paleness of my skin. I usually ran with my back to the sun, but not today. Today I needed to feel it burn into my retinas to wrench from my head some of the painful scenes I had witnessed. I ran across broken shells and felt no pain. I ran until I reached the end of the half-mile strip, and I turned around.

As I turned, I started running as fast as I could down the beach, my feet pounding down the sand, matching the quickening pace of my heart and the increasing tightening across my chest. I began crying as I ran, with my breath coming in even shorter bursts as I hiccupped and sobbed. I realized no one was home. No one was home in Mom's body— her personality and her soul were gone. It was just a body breathing in and out, the urine escaping through the catheter into the bag. "Mom" wasn't really needed to fulfill those functions. It was simply her brain generating that activity.

I started crying harder at these thoughts. Oh, what I wouldn't have given for just one more moment, one more smile, one more nagging phone call, one more "I love you, veeerrrry much." I wished I had listened to her more. I wished I had had more patience. I wished I had given her grandchildren. She had never had a chance to teach me to be a Mom.

Then I literally heard my mom's voice in my head as clear as if she were running alongside beside me: "I just wanted you to be happy, honey, and you didn't have children in this lifetime. As long as you were happy. Besides, I did get that chance," I heard her say.

She drew back the curtain of my mind to reveal a scene that was simultaneously playing out in another dimension. I saw myself sitting on a floral patterned couch, in a sunroom with a white floor. There were two toddlers at my feet, and I was obviously nine months pregnant. My mother was by my side. We were looking through fashion magazines while the kids played. We smiled at each other.

"See, I'm teaching you to be a great Mom." Right then I knew without a doubt that she truly did just want me to be happy—kids or no kids—and that the life I was leading was absolutely perfect. It was such a weird sensation and the entire experience seemed so darned real. To this day, in my bones, I know she was right.

Chapter 54
I Thought You'd Be Interested

walked back and sat in the car, drenched in sweat. Mom would have killed me for sitting in her car against her leather seats all sweaty. I smiled to myself as I grabbed a towel from the trunk and laid it on the seat. As if she'd ever know. "Oh, I know," I heard her say. Great, I thought to myself, now she'll really know everything.

I sat in the car thinking, "Mom is gone. Who am I going to talk to about all of the tiny details of life?" I didn't have the same relationship with my dad as I did with my mom. Dad and I spoke at least once a week for a few minutes. He had a habit of calling me in the middle of my workday from his car while he was stuck in traffic. I didn't have the kind of heart-to-heart talks with him that I did with Mom. Who would

I call to dissect every date and every situation at work? Who would give me advice about things going on with my friends? Dad would never have the patience to listen to all of that girl talk.

Who was going to mail me those random articles from the newspaper about planning for retirement or checking on my health? Mom never told me what to do, but those articles, along with her brief note, "Thought you'd be interested," were very strong suggestions. My dad would never do that, I thought.

As I pulled out of the parking lot to drive back to the condo to shower, I picked up the phone and called my stepmother Patricia.

"Patricia?" I said and started crying again.

"What is it? Did your Mom die? What is going on?" she said very worriedly.

"No, not yet, but I don't think it will be very long. But I have a question to ask you, do you have time for a question?" I could barely talk by this point I was crying so hard.

"I'm having trouble understanding you, but I think you want to ask me a question, is that right?" she asked.

I took a deep breath trying to calm myself so she could understand me.

"Yes. This may seem like a silly question, but once Mom is gone I'm not going to have someone to talk to the way I used to talk to her." I paused, holding back my tears. "Will you be my mom?"

"Of course, honey. Of course I will. I won't ever be able to replace your Mom but I will do the very best I can. You can talk to me about anything," she replied.

"I knew you would say yes. It is kind of a silly question but I felt like I had to ask it. Thank you, Patricia. I love you very much. I'm going to go now because I have to drive."

"You are welcome honey. You call me anytime, anytime at all. I love you, too," she said, and we hung up the phone.

A few months after Mom died, I was facing a really difficult time in a new job. I couldn't get my footing and felt like I was failing all the time. The skills and talent I had built up over the years weren't working in this new situation, and I was at a loss for where to look for help.

My dad happened to call me one Saturday morning as I sat in my kitchen drinking coffee. He was a joker and sometimes came across as a bit gruff, but he had a heart of gold. He'd do anything for me and me for him. We had each other wrapped around our little pinkies. I was lucky to have such a strong male role model in my life.

"Hi Jen, it's Dad, you forgot something," he said.

"Uh oh. He sounds angry," I thought. I hadn't had much sleep the night before because I'd been tossing and turning thinking about work. My nerves were shot.

"What did I forget?" I asked, my throat constricting, fighting back my tears of fear and exhaustion.

"You forgot to call me back," said Dad.

"I'm sorrryyyyyy," I wailed as I burst into deep sobs. I set my coffee cup down on the counter before my shaking hand dropped it.

"What's wrong? What's wrong? Honey, what is going on?"

I could tell he felt guilty because of my reaction. I told him how stressed I had been in the new job and what had happened at work the day before in painstaking detail. He had to ask me to repeat myself from time to time as I was still crying. I don't think I stopped talking for at least 20 minutes, and my dad listened to every single word. Then he did exactly what my mom would have done. He offered some suggestions about management courses I could take, he told me websites to check out, and where I could find other resources. Best of all, he reminded me of how much he loved me and how proud he was of me, just like my mom used to.

I hung up the phone, calm, with a plan of action, and full of love for my dad. I don't think I had ever given him a chance to be there for me that way. I just went to my mom for everything. The reality was my dad had always been there for me, I just hadn't given him the chance. Now I had the opportunity to take our relationship to a new level of connection and intimacy, and I was glad.

A few days later an envelope arrived with my dad's familiar handwriting on the front. I opened it up and out dropped an article on management from the Sunday *New York Times*. The article was wrapped inside a single piece of paper with the simple words, "I thought you'd be interested. Love, Dad," scrawled across the page.

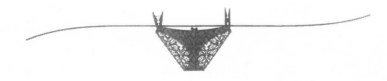

Chapter 55
I Want to Be Alone

I returned to hospice that afternoon and called two of Mom's closet friends to come by to say goodbye. Max and Steve wouldn't be returning. Max was in too much pain and Steve needed to stay to take care of him. Mom hadn't awakened since the previous afternoon, and, after speaking with the nurses, it was clear that she wouldn't be waking up again.

As I sat with Mom during those afternoon hours, watching dusk settle in, I knew in my heart of hearts that she wanted to be alone when she died. She and Max were private people. But more than that, I don't think she would let go if anyone she loved was in the room. She would think it would hurt too much. I called Steve to come over with some suitcases to help me pack up her things.

"Are you sure she'd want us to leave?" he asked me.

"I'm sure. I just get that she is holding on for our sake. Remember how every time one of us kids would enter the room last week she'd awaken and sit up?"

So we packed up her things, taking as much care as she would, folding her clothes ever so carefully, and separating her shoes from her clothes. We left another nightgown and head covering just in case they needed to give her a sponge bath in the next few days. We both walked over to say goodbye, stroking her cheek and kissing her on the forehead. We walked out to go to dinner, and I told Steve that I wouldn't be surprised if we got the call that evening. Sure enough we did. I had dropped him off at the condo along with Mom's suitcases and wasn't in the door five minutes when the phone rang with an unfamiliar Sarasota phone number.

"Jennifer? This is your Mom's nurse. I'm sorry to inform you that your Mom passed away just five minutes ago," she said.

"Thank you for calling. Please do not be sorry. She's not in pain anymore and that is what's important," I replied and hung up the phone.

I called Max, Steve and Aunt Jackie, who would, in turn, inform the rest of the family. I told Teri, who would let the rest of Mom's tap dancing community know. I called my dad and Patricia even though it was hours past their bedtime. Then I got into bed and cried myself to sleep.

Chapter 56
On My Way to Healing

The next day we met with the funeral director to discuss arrangements. While Mom had taken care of most of the arrangements, there were still some small details to be handled, flights to arrange, hotel reservations to make, and an obituary to write and place. It was really difficult to sit with Max, Steve and the funeral director. All of our emotions were heightened and I found myself getting more and more agitated, by what I couldn't precisely put my finger on. It felt like I couldn't get a word in edgewise. For the first time in my life I wanted to scream: "I'm the daughter! I'm the daughter!" I put myself into a timeout and went into my mother's office.

I folded myself into a tiny ball to fit on the loveseat and grabbed a box of tissues. Then I started sobbing while simultaneously blowing my nose. What was going on here? What was my problem? Yes, my mom died, so being emotional was par for the course, but why was I so angry? And at whom? There just wasn't a whole lot of love present. Max wasn't a very emotional guy. "Oh, Mom," I thought to myself, "I just need one of your hugs. I need your love here, I don't have it in me to bring that right now, and I need you Mom. I need a hug. Who is going to give me one of those hugs now?" I started crying harder.

At that precise moment, Max walked in and sat down at the desk chair across from me.

"You giving yourself some space?" he asked. I nodded my head.

"I think that's a good idea. You know, Jen, you can't do everything. A person just can't get everything done in a day. You do realize that," he said and left the room.

As he shut the door I heard my mom's voice as clear as a bell: "There's your hug," my mom said to me. I laughed out loud. Surely, there *was* my hug—it was just Max's style of a hug.

It did get to me, thinking about my mom's choice of men. Neither Max nor my dad was the most effusive guy you'd ever meet. Max was quiet while my dad was boisterous, but neither was the touchy-feely kind. They were both "men's men." Mom was so loving and affectionate. Why would she pick men like that to be with?

I gave it more thought. When Mom first met Max, he had warned her, "Don't you fall in love with me." Mom said she warned him: "Don't you tell me what to do." Later on in their relationship, Max shared his theory that in any relationship there is always someone who loves the other person more. In the beginning it was Mom. At this point, he had told her it was him. Max had definitely expressed his affection for Mom throughout the years—especially by never leaving her side over the last five years. As Golde asked Tevye in Fiddler on the Roof, "If that's not love, what is?"

I wanted that kind of man. I wanted to be in love the way my mom and Max had been. I wanted a man to express his love for me unconditionally—to show me how much he loved me, to share his life with me, and to share his thoughts and dreams with me. My thoughts trailed off and it occurred to me, I had had that kind of man. I was married to that kind of man, but I didn't see it at the time. He loved me unconditionally, but I hadn't been willing to let him love me the way he wanted to. I had never seen things from his eyes. But now I did.

I reached for my phone to call my ex-husband. He had been calling, texting and emailing me over the summer months to let me know that he was there for me and that if I needed anything, I should call him. I had finally sent him an email a few weeks before asking him to stop. I explained that while I appreciated him reaching out, he was not the guy for me right now. I couldn't bring myself to be vulnerable with him. I was too scared that I would get hurt, that he didn't have my best interests at heart, and that, at the end of the day, he had not loved me. After my realization, I now knew he always had.

"Adam, it's me. Mom died last night," I said.

"I'm so sorry, honey," he replied.

"Thanks. We all knew it was coming but it doesn't make it any easier," I said, and added, "I realized something today that I wanted to share with you." I said

I told him what had happened with Max and my thinking about the kind of guy I wanted to be with. "Here is what I realized. All this time I wanted someone to love me unconditionally, and I never realized I had that in you. I just never let you love me the way you wanted to. You are a caretaker and I never let you take care of me. You never got to express yourself fully with me, and I'm really sorry about that. That must have been really difficult for you," I said.

There was a very long pause, and then he chuckled. "You have no idea what a pain in the ass you were."

I laughed along with him. "I know, honey. I'm so sorry."

That conversation was the beginning of our healing process. It led to many more conversations. After a few years, we arrived at a place of peace. When anyone asked why we weren't married, we'd simply say, "We're not married because we're not married. We love each other and we're not married. That's it." No story. No drama. Just the facts ma'am. Life was always simpler that way.

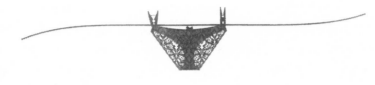

Chapter 57
With Grace And Dignity She Walks

Two days later, Max, Steve and I accompanied my mom's body to Rhode Island for the funeral. My sister-in-law and nephew met us at the airport. Lisa and Aaron were already at the hotel. As I landed, I received a phone call from my best friend, Hallie, who lived only a few hours away. We had known each other for over twenty years. She'd been my Maid of Honor, and I'd be hers.

"Do you want me to come to the funeral with you?" she asked.

I burst into tears. I was so lucky to have her in my life. "Of course," I replied. I thought I might need her to hold me up.

The night before the funeral I sat in my hotel room, fingers poised at the keyboard. I was going to say something to honor my mom the next day, but I was uncertain how to capture everything I wanted to say. How could I put this one woman's life into a few words?

I called my good friend Lars and told him not only did I not know what to write, I was afraid I wouldn't be able to talk. I was afraid I'd get angry, and I was afraid I'd start wailing and clutching my mom's coffin, throwing my body on top of it to keep it from being lowered into the ground. "Okay that last part is just a little dramatic," I admitted.

"What do you want to leave people with?" Lars asked.

"I want to leave people with my mom's grace and dignity. That's the way she lived with her cancer, and that is what inspired people the most," I replied. I smiled and could feel his smile over the telephone.

"Well, there you have it," Lars said chuckling.

I hung up the phone, and the following poem just poured out of me without any thinking on my part. The next day, I read it at the funeral.

With Grace and Dignity She Walks

With grace and dignity she walked, she sauntered, she entered a room, really, captivating anyone who was in her presence with her quiet beauty, intelligence and thirst for knowledge about everything and everyone.

With grace and dignity she listened—to music, the sound of her husband's chuckle, the sound of her children playing music, the laughter of her grandchildren;

With grace and dignity she listened to the words of loved ones, holding those moments dear, offering heartfelt advice, her heart bigger than the Milky Way—carrying so very much love;

With grace and dignity she spoke, eloquently defending her dissertation, teaching children, teaching teachers, teaching piano, teaching tap dance—so patient, so kind, so tender;

With grace and dignity she inspired each of us to hold every moment dear, to go for our dreams, to pick ourselves up and dust ourselves off when we failed—her belief in us often bigger than our belief in ourselves.

With grace and dignity she lived, right up until the very end, on her own terms, squeezing every ounce of life out of life, all of us in awe of her strength, her beauty, her gentleness;

With grace and dignity and love we remember her, free now of the body which imprisoned her;

With grace and dignity she now walks;

Starlit, moonlight serenading ocean breezes filling the air as she tap dances along the shoreline,

Arms raised overhead, dancing between the waves, taking her final bow, her final curtain call. — September 18, 2011

I read the poem at the funeral, with my best friend holding me up as I sobbed my way through it. Max received a framed copy from one of his friends down in Florida. He called me after he got it: "Coken? Did you read this at the funeral?" he asked. I sure did I told him. "I don't know how you do it? You have such a way with words," he said. He didn't remember a word, but loved it so much that he kept a framed copy on their piano.

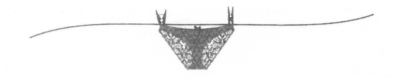

Chapter 58
I Wouldn't Change A Thing

*M*onths passed. Milestones passed—Mom's birthday, Christmas, her wedding anniversary, my resignation from my job, my moving in with a friend to figure out what was next for me given I had just moved 2,000 miles for the job in the first place.

An old friend called. We hadn't spoken in at least a year. I told him about Mom's passing. As many people do, he kept repeating, "I'm so sorry. I'm so sorry, Jen." I know what he said was truly from his heart, as it was for so many others. But for the first time, I responded out loud, "I'm not sorry, Ross. I wouldn't change a thing."

I'm not sorry that Mom is out of her body because she was in so much pain. To see someone so vibrant go from a size eight to a size zero, someone who had to buy big shirts to cover up her swollen belly was horrible.

I am sorry she died so young. I would have given anything to have her with me another twenty-three years. I was again reminded that my grandmother lived to be ninety-four—Mom was only seventy-one when she died.

But would I change the fact that she died? Yes. Who wouldn't? But I'd only want her around for the next twenty-three years if I could retain all of the wisdom I gained from being with her as she transitioned. I'd only change things if I could retain all of the lessons I have learned about life, love and myself during the days and months after she passed.

I was going through her things the month after she died. Max was adamant about getting her things out of the house because he couldn't bear the pain of seeing them. I went through her jewelry, sorted and gave away shoes and clothes to friends and sent some to family. I put her wigs and hats in a special bag for the American Cancer Society. I made certain to take for myself all of the fancy underwear she had made me promise to take.

(For the record, I continue to wear my mom's thong underwear because Hanky Panky's are the most comfortable thong I've ever worn. As hers wear out, I spend the twenty dollars to replace each pair. There isn't a day goes by that I'm not wearing the panties and thinking of her, and her seventy-one-year-old ass in them. It's like our little secret.)

I sorted out all of her paperwork. I threw away all the spiral notebooks where she kept every detail of her cancer treatment over the previous five years. Her neat tiny handwriting outlined how she felt, the food she ate, how much she weighed, test results and snippets of conversations she had had. I hesitated for a moment, wondering what I might be missing in the pages. But I couldn't bear to re-live every single day, so out they went.

I was going through folders of her theater performances. All of her reviews were there —the good, the bad and some truly ugly. A few were scathing; I think I would have crumbled and given up. Yet, my mother kept performing. She didn't let one person's opinion hold her back from what she wanted to do. She so believed in herself. I didn't know that about her. I always thought she was so sensitive. Obviously, I was mistaken.

I, on the other hand, often feel like a feather in the wind. One thoughtless unkind word or one look misinterpreted could send me off the deep end of making myself wrong, trying to figure out what was wrong with me, and losing confidence nearly immediately.

I often thought of her as wound too tightly, so many times she wouldn't say anything, bite her tongue and lash out later on. I assumed my interpretation of her was correct and that she ought to learn to say what is on her mind more. Certainly she was naive to think that people had good motives all the time.

I think however, I was the naive one. At my core, I often assumed the worst of others, didn't trust people, kept at least a little bit of my heart walled off and protected—all the while pretending that I loved unconditionally. But I didn't. The bottomless well of love that my mom had for others was absolutely astounding. I have learned this lesson from her—to love is to accept unconditionally and to be with someone just as they are and just as they are not.

My mother had an iron will, and I never truly saw this until she made certain that she had tried every single possible cure or treatment for her cancer. She wanted nothing left on the table. In the end, she was at peace when she died. She was ready to go because she had exhausted every option. From her, I learned to do deal with reality with grace and dignity, to get my questions answered, to leave no stone unturned, and to walk away knowing I had given it my all. In the end, it was she who had "failed" spectacularly.

When my mother told the doctor that she didn't have a bucket list, I was shocked. For whatever reason, I never thought my mom was fulfilled. I never thought she was leading the life she wanted to lead. It felt like she had to give up so very much to be there for us kids and to provide for us. That wasn't true at all.

She may have had to give up some things at certain times, but she gave up those things because she chose to give up those things. There was nothing my mother did that she did not want to do, and there was nothing she didn't do that she did want to do. She had a great job that provided security for her family. She saved money for retirement and for other things. She performed.

I used to say that I was very much like my dad, an entrepreneur, big personality, quick to anger but someone who doesn't play it safe. I rebelled against how I thought my mom was. But my mom was extraordinarily smart. She built her life in a way that allowed her to have everything. She had the great love of her life. She had a great career and great friends. She had it all.

See, if my mom were still alive, I would continue to see the illusion I had built up in front of me. So, would I change her dying? Only, if I could retain all of the life lessons that I learned from her dying, and I know you can't have it both ways.

Don't get me wrong. I do have regrets. I regret not picking up the phone more often when I thought of her. I regret losing my patience at times, and talking to her in a way that I'm certain left her feeling dumb. I regret any arguments we ever had when I was an adult daughter. I regret not listening more. Not asking for her advice more. Not taking her advice more. I regret it all.

But in the end, I wouldn't change any of it because we had the relationship we had to learn what we each had to learn in this lifetime. We chose each other. I chose this amazing woman to be my mother to be able to experience what death would be like, and experience the impact on my own life. My mom's dying prepared me for my own inevitable death, but mostly it reminded me to create a beautiful life for myself, right now and not hold back, play it safe and wait for everything to "turn out."

Epilogue

Dear Reader,

Since I finished writing this book, I've spent a lot of time reflecting on what I learned during the time that my mom died and my marriage ended. For any of us, losing a loved one is challenging and sometimes we don't think we'll get through it. We feel we are at our max and hope that life doesn't throw us any more curve balls. But 2011 seemed to be the year of curve balls. While dealing with my mom's death, I also was facing the end of my marriage (another death). Then eleven other people in my life died out of the blue – some of whom I was very close to and others I was not, but all were shocking. While all of this was going on, I moved back to DC after being gone eight years (leaving my support structure) to take a new job I was really excited about. However, after only five months I realized the new position wasn't a good fit for where I was at in my life so I wound up leaving. At the time I was living in a company apartment while I waited for my new home to be built. Once I left I no longer had the income to support the new home. (Thankfully I had a terrific realtor and friend who made it possible for me to resell the home before I even stepped foot in the door.)

I have coached thousands of people over the last eighteen years and I can tell you that any ONE of these events would've left a human being hiding under their proverbial covers. That's what we human beings do when facing dire circumstances – we figure out some way to numb ourselves. For some that may be eating or drinking to excess; for others it may be burying themselves in their work; for others it may be completely disconnecting and becoming a recluse; and for others it may be trying to control everything in their lives in some way, shape or form.

No matter who you are, you find a way to cope with the circumstances of your life.

But I'm not interested in you coping with life – coping comes with some degree of suffering or struggle or both. I'm interested in you being complete. What do I mean by that? To be able to be with any of the circumstances of your life – no matter how horrific – and be able to say with complete and total authenticity that you wouldn't change a thing because you learned and you grew.

So in that vein, below I've outlined what I learned from my adventures with life. I hope that by adopting some or all of these lessons you too will find yourself learning and growing. I'd also whole-heartedly recommend anyone and everyone doing the Landmark Forum (www.landmarkworldwide.com). That one single weekend will completely alter what you think is possible for your life, what you think you are capable of and what the future holds for you. I couldn't have accomplished the breakthroughs I had without that training. But that choice is wholly in your hands. (And no, I don't get any money or a new toaster if you register.)

LESSON ONE: Do not turn away from the hard stuff – as much as you may want to. Experience everything, don't shove it away. Move through it, don't eat it. Have the tough conversations with yourself and others. Sometimes you have to do that moment by moment by moment. Just grab those snarling dogs by the ears and look them straight in their eyes. Confront every aspect of yourself that you don't want to see because you are committed to being complete.

LESSON TWO: Don't numb yourself. Do not check out (drugs, alcohol, shopping trips, burying yourself in your work etc.) This will require you to be more courageous than you've ever had to be in your entire life. I'm not asking you to do something I haven't already done. Listen, if you don't deal with what is happening now you WILL deal with it at some point. If you don't deal with your emotions, all of the "what ifs," the "how abouts," the "why nots" now, they will all come up to bite you in the butt down the road. So no time like the present, right?

LESSON THREE: Create community. When human beings are dealing with tough stuff we usually don't want to burden anyone else. But guess what? People love supporting their friends and family in need but we so rarely get to because we're all trying to be brave and not burden each other. Don't you love being that shoulder for your friends? Well they love doing that for you too. This won't always be easy. It will require you to get out of your comfort zone, be vulnerable and tell someone the intimate details of what is really going on with you.

Saying everything is important for two reasons. First, if you don't tell the truth, your friends won't know how to support you. You may not know what you need to feel supported, let them make suggestions and see what works for you. Second, you want to get it out of that space between your ears that's been keeping you up at night. Many times when I say things out loud that I've been thinking I realize it isn't as dramatic as I've made it out to be, or I find a solution in the conversation.

Finally, you may experience shame or embarrassment – especially if you've been trying to hold it together or have always been the strong one. Please realize this. Any human being on the planet who is dealing with what you are dealing with would likely be feeling those same feelings, or having the same thoughts or taking the same actions. You are not alone. Thousands of people have been down the path you are on and each has found his or her way out.

LESSON FOUR: Don't be a victim. Blaming your circumstances will do you no good because while you likely will craft a lovely explanation for why life sucks at the moment it will make absolutely no difference and continue to leave you powerless. So, put on your big girl or big boy panties and look within and ask yourself: What am I holding on to that I can let go of? Have you ever heard the story about how trappers catch monkeys in the jungle? First they cut a hole in a box big enough only for a monkey's arm or a banana but not both. Then they put the bananas inside the box. A monkey comes along and grabs the banana but can't get its hand and the banana, out of the box. The monkey will stay with its arm inside the box because it won't let go of the banana – sacrificing its own freedom. Human beings are the same way. We'd rather sacrifice our own freedom and hold on to things that aren't serving us instead of letting go. Put down the banana!

Here is another empowering question to ask yourself: What do I resent about what is happening in this situation that I am willing to let go of? The definition of resentment is the "feeling or displeasure or indignation at some act, remark, person, etc. regarded as causing injury or insult." Look, maybe someone did intentionally set out to cause you displeasure or indignation – that is for them to deal with. Don't you give away your power by continuing to be angry at the person or situation. The only one harmed by you holding on to your resentment is you.

Here are a few more great questions to ask: What did I step over or ignore that led to this circumstance? Where did I comprise my values and give into something I knew wasn't right for me or my life? This stepping over question is a big one. Stepping over something is like stepping over the dog poop in your back yard. The more you leave it, the less room your dog has for running around. Stepping over issues in our lives is the same kind of thing. The more you step over the less freedom you experience to be yourself and express yourself.

LESSON FIVE: Don't Get Stuck With Why Me? When the you know what hits the fan every single human being asks "why me?" It's natural. So ask it, but don't get stuck with it because there is "no cheese down that tunnel." I hereby give you permission to have it over for dinner and have a few drinks with it, but don't let it sleep in your bed because you will regret it in the morning. See, going to sleep with that question is not only going to color your waking moments but your dreaming moments as well. It will become embedded in your brain as a new neuronal pathway. Upon awakening, what was merely a question blurted out last night in a fit of rage by an upset five year-old having a tantrum (yes I mean you and it takes one to know one) has now become a part of "you." You'll forget it was merely one thought (among many) and it will now become a part of your new reality. So, here's a better question to ask – what can I learn from what is happening around me?

LESSON SIX: You will survive. Seriously. You will. It may not seem like it at the time. Life may seem so much bigger than you are, but it isn't. I'm sure you've had at least ONE other experience in life where it felt like all hell was breaking loose and you'd never get over it. Think about it. Take a minute and think back over all the years you have lived and bring one event to mind that seemed completely overwhelming. Got it? Good. If you survived that part of life, you will survive this one. I'm of the belief that absolutely everything that comes your way is meant to teach you about you; that we choose our path before we incarnate. From this belief system, every circumstance you are dealing with and every person you come into contact with (yep even that person) is here to teach you something. The question is what lesson are you learning?

Afterword

The following material is reprinted with permission from the Ovarian Cancer National Alliance website (www.ovariancancer.org).

What is Ovarian Cancer?

Ovarian cancer is a growth of abnormal malignant cells that begins in the ovaries (women's reproductive glands that produce ova). Cancer that spreads to the ovaries but originates at another site is not considered ovarian cancer.

Ovarian tumors can be benign (noncancerous) or malignant (cancerous). Although abnormal, cells of benign tumors do not metastasize (spread to other parts of the body). Malignant cancer cells in the ovaries can metastasize in two ways:

- Directly to other organs in the pelvis and abdomen (the more common way)
- Through the bloodstream or lymph nodes to other parts of the body

While the causes of ovarian cancer are unknown, some theories exist:

- Genetic errors may occur because of the repeated "wear and tear" of the monthly release of an egg.
- Increased hormone levels before and during ovulation may stimulate the growth of abnormal cells.

Statistics

In the United States, doctors must report any diagnosis of cancer to a state registry. The federal government, through the Centers for Disease Control and Prevention's National Program of Cancer Registries, oversees the registries in 45 states, the District of Columbia, and three territories. The Surveillance, Epidemiology and End Results (SEER) Program of the National Cancer Institute funds the remaining five statewide cancer registries. Together, the two programs cover the country's population.

The following statistics come primarily from the most recent findings of the Surveillance, Epidemiology and End Results (SEER) Program of the National Cancer Institute. SEER numbers are age-adjusted and based on actual data; SEER data is available for most data through 2008. More recent statistics, such as 2012 incidence numbers, are projections from the American Cancer Society.

The American Cancer Society estimates that in 2012, about 22,280 new cases of ovarian cancer will be diagnosed and 15,500 women will die of ovarian cancer in the United States.

According to the data, the mortality rates for ovarian cancer have not improved in forty years since the "War on Cancer" was declared. However, other cancers have shown a marked reduction in mortality, due to the availability of early detection tests and improved treatments. Unfortunately, this is not the case with ovarian cancer, which is still the deadliest of all gynecologic cancers.

The Surveillance, Epidemiology and End Results (SEER) Program reports that on January 1, 2008 in the United States approximately 177,578 women were alive who had been diagnosed with ovarian cancer (including those who had been cured of the disease).

Year	Incidence	Deaths
1999	19,676	13,627
2000	19,672	14,060
2001	19,719	14,414
2002	19,792	14,682
2003	20,445	14,657
2004	20,069	14,716
2005	19,842	14,787
2006	19,994	14,487
2007	20,749	14,621
2008 (Projected)	21,650	15,520
2009 (Projected)	21,550	14,600
2010 (Projected)	21,880	13,850
2011 (Projected)	21,990	15,460

Ovarian cancer accounts for approximately three percent of cancers in women. While the ninth most common cancer among women, ovarian cancer is the fifth leading cause of cancer-related death among women, and is the deadliest of gynecologic cancers. Mortality rates are slightly higher for Caucasian women than for African-American women.[1]

A Woman's Lifetime Risk:

A woman's lifetime risk of developing invasive ovarian cancer is 1 in 71. A woman's lifetime risk of dying from invasive ovarian cancer is 1 in 95.

Age:

Approximately 1.2 percent were diagnosed under age 20; 3.5 percent between 20 and 34; 7.3 percent between 35 and 44; 19.1 percent between 45 and 54; 23.1 percent between 55 and 64; 19.7 percent between 65 and 74; 18.2 percent between 75 and 84; and 8.0 percent 85+ years of age.

Approximate Age at Diagnosis: FY2002-2006

Age Diagnosed

● Under 20 ● 20-34 ● 35-44 ● 45-54 ● 55-64 ● 65-74
● 85 & older ● 75-84

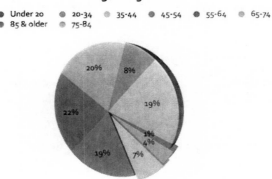

From 2002 to 2008, the median age at diagnosis was 63. From 2003 to 2007, the median age at death from ovarian cancer was 71.

Survival:

Survival Rate and Diagnosis for Varied Stages (1999-2005)

Stage at diagnosis	Five-year relative Survival Rate	Percentage of Total Women Diagnosed
Localized (cancer is limited to organ from which is originated)	93.8	15 percent
Regional (cancer is spread to nearby lymph nodes or organs and tissue)	72.8	17 percent
Distant (cancer has spread to distant organs or lymph nodes	28.2	62 percent
Unstaged (not enough information to identify a stage)	27.3	7 percent

Ovarian cancer survival rates are much lower than other cancers that affect women.

- The relative five-year survival rate is 46 percent. Survival rates vary depending on the stage of diagnosis.
- Women diagnosed at an early stage have a much higher five-year survival rate than those diagnosed at a later stage.
- Approximately 15 percent of ovarian cancer patients are diagnosed early.[2]

Risk Factors

While most women with ovarian cancer do not have any known risk factors, some do exist. If a woman has one or more risk factors, she will not necessarily develop ovarian cancer; however, her risk may be higher than the average woman's.

Genetics

About 10 to 15 percent of women diagnosed with ovarian cancer have a hereditary tendency to develop the disease. The most significant risk factor for ovarian cancer is an inherited genetic mutation in one of two genes: breast cancer gene 1 (BRCA1) or breast cancer gene 2 (BRCA2). These genes are responsible for about 5 to 10 percent of all ovarian cancers.

Eastern European women and women of Ashkenazi Jewish descent are at a higher risk of carrying BRCA1 and BRCA2 mutations.

Since these genes are linked to both breast and ovarian cancer, women who have had breast cancer have an increased risk of ovarian cancer.

Another known genetic link to ovarian cancer is an inherited syndrome called hereditary nonpolyposis colorectal cancer (HNPCC or Lynch Syndrome). While HNPCC poses the greatest risk of colon cancer, women with HNPCC have about a 12 percent lifetime risk of developing ovarian cancer.

Women who have one first-degree relative with ovarian cancer but no known genetic mutation still have an increased risk of developing ovarian cancer. The lifetime risk of a woman who has a first degree relative with ovarian cancer is five percent (the average woman's lifetime risk is 1.4 percent).

Increasing Age

All women are at risk of developing ovarian cancer regardless of age; however, a woman's risk is highest during her 60s and increases with age through her late 70s. About 69 percent of women diagnosed with ovarian cancer in the United States from 2002 to 2006 were 55 or older. The median age (at which half of all reported cases are older and half are younger) at diagnosis is 63.

Reproductive History and Infertility

Research suggests a relationship between the number of menstrual cycles in a woman's lifetime and her risk of developing ovarian cancer. A woman is at an increased risk if she:

- Started menstruating at an early age (before 12),
- Has not given birth to any children,
- Had her first child after 30,
- Experienced menopause after 50,
- Has never taken oral contraceptives,
- Infertility, regardless of whether or not a woman uses fertility drugs, also increases the risk of ovarian cancer.

Hormone Replacement Therapy

Doctors may prescribe hormone replacement therapy to alleviate symptoms associated with menopause (hot flashes, night sweats, sleeplessness, vaginal dryness) that occur as the body adjusts to decreased levels of estrogen. Hormone replacement therapy usually involves treatment with either estrogen alone (for women who have had a hysterectomy) or a combination of estrogen with progesterone or progestin (for women who have not had a hysterectomy).

Women who use menopausal hormone therapy are at an increased risk for ovarian cancer. Recent studies indicate that using a combination of estrogen and progestin for five or more years significantly increases the risk of ovarian cancer in women who have not had a hysterectomy. Ten or more years of estrogen use increases the risk of ovarian cancer in women who have had a hysterectomy.

Obesity

Various studies have found a link between obesity and ovarian cancer. A 2009 study found that obesity was associated with an almost 80 percent higher risk of ovarian cancer in women 50 to 71 who had not taken hormones after menopause.

Reducing Risk

Women can reduce the risk of developing ovarian cancer in many ways; however, there is no prevention method for the disease. All women are at risk because ovarian cancer does not strike only one ethnic or age group. A healthcare professional can help a woman identify ways to reduce her risk as well as decide if consultation with a genetic counselor is appropriate.

Oral Contraceptives (birth control pills)

The use of oral contraceptives decreases the risk of developing ovarian cancer, especially when used for several years. Women who use oral contraceptives for five or more years have about a 50 percent lower risk of developing ovarian cancer than women who have never used oral contraceptives.

Symptoms of Ovarian Cancer

For years, women have known that ovarian cancer was not the silent killer it was said to be. Over the past decade, science has confirmed what women have long known: ovarian cancer has symptoms.

The symptoms are:

- Bloating
- Pelvic or abdominal pain
- Difficulty eating or feeling full quickly
- Urinary symptoms (urgency or frequency)

As medical research continues to investigate this important issue, numerous studies have been published indicating that symptoms may not occur until late stage or that they may not improve health outcomes. The Ovarian Cancer National Alliance believes that symptoms are still relevant, but they are not a definitive diagnostic tool. Since there is no diagnostic tool for ovarian cancer, symptom awareness remains of key importance. Being cognizant of symptoms can help women get diagnosed sooner.

Women with ovarian cancer report that symptoms are persistent and represent a change from normal for their bodies. The frequency and/or number of such symptoms are key factors in the diagnosis of ovarian cancer. Several studies show that even early stage ovarian cancer can produce these symptoms.

Women who have these symptoms almost daily for more than a few weeks should see their doctor, preferably a gynecologist. Prompt medical evaluation may lead to detection at the earliest possible stage of the disease. Early stage diagnosis is associated with an improved prognosis.

Several other symptoms have been commonly reported by women with ovarian cancer. These symptoms include: fatigue, indigestion, back pain, pain with intercourse, constipation and menstrual irregularities. However, these other symptoms are not as useful in identifying ovarian cancer because they are also found in equal frequency in women in the general population who do not have ovarian cancer.

The Ovarian Cancer National Alliance offers two free resources women can use to track symptoms of ovarian cancer: an Ovarian Cancer Symptom Diary App (http://www.ovariancancer.org/app/ and a printable Symptom Diary (http://www.ovariancancer.org/resources/diary/).

EARLY DETECTION

Early detection of ovarian cancer saves women's lives. No screening test exists that can test all women for ovarian cancer. The Pap test does not test for ovarian cancer; it screens for cervical cancer.

Not only do researchers need to develop an early detection test for ovarian cancer, like mammograms for breast cancer and Pap tests for cervical cancer, but also women and medical professionals need to become more aware of ovarian cancer symptoms.

While no early detection tool exists for all women, several tests exist for women who are at a high risk. If a woman has ovarian cancer symptoms, a strong family history, or a genetic predisposition such as a BRCA mutation, doctors may monitor her with one of three tests or a combination of them:

Blood Test

The protein CA-125 exists in greater concentration in cancerous cells. Though a high count of this protein may help doctors identify ovarian cancer, premenopausal women may have an elevated CA-125 due to benign conditions unrelated to ovarian cancer. Uterine fibroids, liver disease, inflammation of the fallopian tubes, and other types of cancer can raise a woman's CA-125 level, often causing a false positive test for ovarian cancer.

Although the CA-125 blood test is more accurate in postmenopausal women, it is not a reliable early detection test for ovarian cancer. In about 20 percent of advanced stage ovarian cancer cases and 50 percent of early stage cases, the CA-125 is not elevated even though ovarian cancer is present. As a result, doctors generally use the CA-125 blood test in combination with a transvaginal ultrasound.

The CA-125 blood test can be an important tool for evaluating the disease's progress and tumors' response to treatment. Additionally, this test can monitor a woman's CA-125 level for evidence of recurrence.

OVA1 has also been approved by the Food and Drug Administration (FDA) for risk stratification. A woman who presents with a known tumor may have this test to determine if her surgery should be done by a gynecologist or a gynecologic oncologist – doctors who are specially trained to treat women with gynecologic cancers.

Transvaginal Ultrasound

- A transvaginal ultrasound is a test used to examine a woman's reproductive organs and bladder.
- To administer the test, the doctor inserts a probe into the woman's vagina. The probe sends off sound waves which reflect off body structures. The waves are then received by a computer that turns them into a picture.

Pelvic Exam

- A pelvic exam should be a part of a woman's regular female health exam.
- This exam requires the doctor to place one or two fingers into a woman's vagina and another over her abdomen to feel the size, shape, and position of the ovaries and uterus. Ovarian cancer is rarely detected in a pelvic exam and usually in an advanced stage if it is.

DIAGNOSIS

If a woman has the signs and symptoms of ovarian cancer, her doctor will probably perform a complete pelvic exam, a transvaginal or pelvic ultrasound, and a CA-125 blood test. Used individually, these tests are not definitive; they are most effective when used in combination with each other. Doctors may also use a CT scan or PET scan as part of the diagnostic process. The only definitive way to determine if a patient has ovarian cancer is through surgery and biopsy.

Gynecologic Oncologist

Multiple studies conducted over the past decade have shown that an ovarian cancer patient's chance of survival is significantly improved when her surgery is performed by a gynecologic oncologist. One analysis of multiple studies found that women whose surgeries were performed by gynecologic oncologists had a median survival time that was 50 percent greater than women whose surgeries were done by general gynecologists or other surgeons inexperienced in optimal debulking procedures. Sometimes referred to as cytoreductive surgery, debulking involves removal of as much of the tumor as possible.

As part of the debulking procedure, doctors try to stage definitively the disease and identify the optimal treatment for the cancer. Proper staging and optimal debulking translate into improved overall survival for women at any stage of ovarian cancer.

Gynecologic oncologists have greater success in treating ovarian cancer as a result of their tendency to perform more aggressive surgery. Women whose tumors have been reduced to less than one centimeter have a better response to chemotherapy and improved survival rate. Gynecologic oncologists also are more likely to perform the multiple peritoneal and lymph node biopsies necessary to ensure adequate surgical staging.

The Women's Cancer Network has a "Find a Doctor" feature on its Web site (www.wcn.org) where visitors can search for gynecologic oncologists by ZIP code. Women can also find the nearest gynecologic oncologist by calling (800) 444-4441.

Recurrence

When cancer returns after a period of remission, it is considered a recurrence. A cancer recurrence happens because some cancer cells were left behind and eventually grow and become apparent. The cancer may come back to the same place as the original tumor or to another place in the body. Around 70 percent of patients diagnosed with ovarian cancer will have a recurrence.

One of the factors in determining a patient's risk of recurrence is the stage of the cancer at diagnosis:

- Patients diagnosed in stage I have a 10 percent chance of recurrence.
- Patients diagnosed in stage II have a 30 percent chance of recurrence.
- Patients diagnosed in stage III have a 70 to 90 percent chance of recurrence.
- Patients diagnosed in stage IV have a 90 to 95 percent chance of recurrence.

Recurrent ovarian cancer is treatable but rarely curable. Women with recurrent ovarian cancer may have to undergo another surgery. Because many women with recurrent ovarian cancer receive chemotherapy for a prolonged period of time, sometimes continuously, the toxicities of therapy are a major factor in treatment decisions.

The effectiveness and type of treatment for recurrent ovarian cancer depends on what kind of chemotherapy the patient received in the past, the side effects associated with previous treatments, the length of time since finishing the previous treatment, and the extent of the recurrent cancer. Chemotherapy is used to stop the progression of cancer and prolong the patient's survival. Sometimes, surgery is used to relieve symptoms, such as a blocked bowel caused by the recurrence.

A woman, in consultation with her doctor, should set realistic goals for what to expect from treatment. This may mean weighing the possible positive outcomes of a new treatment against the possible negative ones. At some point, a woman may decide that continuing treatment is unlikely to improve her health or survival. A woman must be certain that she is comfortable with her decision whatever it is.

WITHDRAWN
WITHDRAWN

CPSIA information can be obtained
at www.ICGtesting.com
Printed in the USA
LVOW11s1707290117
522483LV00045B/125/P